MEDICINES MANAGEMENT FOR RESIDENTIAL AND NURSING HOMES

A toolkit for best practice and accredited learning

Roy Lilley and Paul Lambden
with Alan Gillies

Radcliffe Publishing
Oxford • Seattle

Radcliffe Publishing Ltd
18 Marcham Road
Abingdon
Oxon OX14 1AA
United Kingdom

www.radcliffe-oxford.com
Electronic catalogue and worldwide online ordering facility.

© 2007 Roy Lilley and Paul Lambden

British Library Cataloguing in Publication Data

A catalogue record for this book is available from the British Library.

ISBN-10 1 84619 120 3
ISBN-13 978 1 84619 120 6

Typeset by Anne Joshua & Associates, Oxford
Printed and bound by TJ International Ltd, Padstow, Cornwall

CONTENTS

ABOUT THE AUTHORS

Roy Lilley is a former NHS Trust chairman who now writes and broadcasts on NHS and health issues. He is the originator of the top-selling Tool-Kit series of books.

Dr Paul Lambden BSc MB BS BDS FDSRCS MRCS DRCOG MHSM
Paul is a doctor and a dentist with a degree in pharmacology. Following 15 years in medical and dental practice he became an NHS Trust chief executive and subsequently worked as chairman and chief executive of a charity, then for a local medical committee and more recently in the medical defence industry. He was formerly a special adviser to the Parliamentary Health Select Committee. He now works, part-time, in general practice, teaching and in the medical defence arena.

Alan Gillies Alan Gillies is Professor of Information Management at the University of Central Lancashire. He developed the University's first complete Masters programme to be delivered by e-learning in 2000, and is head of health informatics. He is a Fellow of the British Computing Society, and holds an honorary doctorate from a medical University in Transylvania.

His most recent book title was *The Clinicians Guide to Surviving IT*.

ACKNOWLEDGEMENTS

Yasmin Ashraf from Grace Muriel House, St Albans Hertfordshire, for her invaluable technical advice and practical experience. The Royal College of Nursing: their excellent website is full of good-stuff (www.rcn.org.uk/). Department of Health (www.doh.gov.uk). Royal Pharmaceutical Society of Great Britain (www.rpsgb.org.uk). The Commission for Social Care Inspection (www.csci.org.uk). BBC (www.bbc.co.uk). Boots – a very useful and informative website and excellent pharmacy systems (www.boots.com/microsites/microsite_info_template.jsp?contentId=3417).

DEDICATION

For Paula, who is for me absolutely the right prescription (PL) and for SSL, who is trying to decide if I am the right prescription (RL).

INTRODUCTION

In February 2006 the BBC's excellent health news website (news.bbc.co.uk/ 1/hi/health/default.stm) carried a story, following a report from the Commission for Social Care Inspection, about the standard of medicines management in residential care homes.

Here are some extracts from the report by Hannah Goff, the BBC's health reporter:

Why care home drug errors happen

When inspectors said thousands of care home residents were being given the wrong medication – the image of a grotty, poorly run nursing home reared its stereotypical head.

How could something so simple as giving a patient their daily dose of tablets be going so wrong, so many times over?

But according to care professionals, management of residents' medication is one of the most complex areas of running a nursing home.

And unless failsafe practices are adhered to, the results can be very damaging to both the resident and the care worker.

In the case of a care or nursing home resident, there are so many more people inputting into the system.

The prescription might be written by a GP or consultant.

The pharmacist then has to make it up, then it will go to the staff in the home for storage and then a number of different people may be involved in the issuing the medication to patients.

Adrian Webb, who runs a specialist mental health unit for elderly mentally ill people in central Manchester, says the main problem is that there are so many people in the chain.

An ordinary patient would take their GP's prescription to the pharmacist and then, presumably, take the medication in the advised dose.

Mr Webb, who is a registered nurse and oversees the distribution of drugs in the Victoria Park Nursing Home, says: 'At each stage of the process there is potential for error. It has been known for prescriptions to come from doctors that are incorrect. But it's very easy for someone to type 100 instead of 10, for example.'

The report went on to raise some very worrying issues.

Clearly, it's time to sort this out!

In medicines management there are 4 'rights':

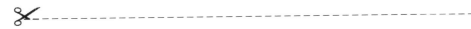

> # The right medicine in the right dose, for the right patient at the right time.

That's the aim of this book . . .

. . . and it should be your aim too. Rip this page out and stick it on the wall where the medicines are stored. It can't do any harm as a reminder!

HOW TO GET THE BEST FROM THIS BOOK

Relax! This is not a book you have to read from cover to cover. It's not designed that way.

It would be nice if you did sit down and gallop through all the pages but we know that no one has time for that. If you want to get all the questions and exercises right, you will, eventually, have to have gone through the book, thoroughly.

However, for now, it isn't necessary. Flip through the pages and have a look. You will find a series of checklists, to-do lists, ideas, tips and warnings. And, there is a fair amount of duplication.

So, here's how it works. The first part of the book is a summary, for the fast readers who need to get an overview of safe medicines management. The rest of the book looks at the issues in more detail. It goes into some of the issues in greater depth.

Throughout you will find questions and exercises that you can complete, on your own, as part of a learning exercise with the people you work with, as a framework for teaching, or online to achieve your learning accreditation.

There are a number of symbols. Here's what they mean.

✂ Something to cut out or copy. It drives the publisher barmy, but we don't care!

☺ Good stuff to know or do.

☹ You'll not want to screw this up.

😐 Mmmmm . . .

☑ Get a tick in the box and you've got it right.

Definitely bad, a hazard, a warning and death if you get it wrong.

 A 'must get right'.

 Make a note or try an exercise.

 Something to do with IT, computers and that type of stuff.

 Read this carefully . . .

 Against the clock, or take time to think, or something to do with timing.

 Obvious, isn't it?

 Data and numbers and stuff like that.

 And there is one of these – to flag something up. Can you find it?

 Take time out for an exercise.

Finally, at the end of the book there is some stuff that doctors and nurses know – that you might find useful to know, too.

OK, got all that?

ACCREDITED LEARNING

For information about a wide range of online supporting resources, including questions and exercises that you can complete at your own pace, submit for assessment and have your learning accredited, go to

www.radcliffe-oxford.com/carehomesmedicine.

SECTION ONE: INTRODUCTION

This book is a distillation of common sense, good practice and an overview of the regulations; it is not designed to be the Gold Standard, or 'the only way', or the 'approved way' but it is a good foundation for you to build your own good practice and try and do even better than the suggestions in the book.

Rules and regulations? Here are the some of the main regulations, codes of practice, organisations and Acts of Parliament that cover the management of medicines in UK residential homes:

- Pharmaceutical Services to Nursing Homes (1990)
- The Administration and Control of Medicines in Residential and Children's Homes (1994)
- The Administration and Control of Medicines in Care Homes (2001)
- Medicines, Ethics and Practice: A Guide for Pharmacists
- The Care Standards Act 2000 and the Regulation of Care (Scotland) Act 2001
- The National Care Standards Commission for England (NCSC)
- The Care Standards Inspectorate for Wales (CSIW)
- The Scottish Commission for the Regulation of Care (SCRC) – Care Commission
- Nursing and Midwifery Council (NMC)
- The General Social Care Council for England
- The General Social Care Council for Wales
- The Scottish Social Services Council
- The Medicines Act 1968
- The Misuse of Drugs Act 1971
- The Misuse of Drugs (Safe Custody) Regulations 1973 SI 1973 No 798 as amended by Misuse of Drugs Regulations 2001
- The NHS Scotland Pharmaceutical Service (Regulations) 1995
- The Social Work (Scotland) Act 1968 as amended by The Regulation of Care Act 2001
- The Children's Act 1995 and 2001
- The Data Protection Act 1998
- The Care Standards Act 2000
- The Regulation of Care (Scotland) Act 2001
- The Health and Social Care Act 2001
- . . . and probably a lot more that we've missed!
  . . . some bedtime reading for you!

Just in case that doesn't excite you, this book should give you a feel for what good, safe, medicines practice is all about.

HERE'S THE BAD NEWS

In March 2004, the National Care Standards Commission (NCSC), a predecessor organisation to the Commission for Social Care Inspection (CSCI) (www.csci.org.uk/), reported on homes' performance on managing medication. The report identified:

> . . . significant deficiencies in homes' performance and practice and was instrumental in focusing attention on the need for homes to take urgent remedial action.

What they were most concerned about was:

The wrong medication being given to residents

There was evidence of:

- poor recording of medicines received and administered;
- medicines being inappropriately handled by unqualified staff;
- medicines being stored inappropriately.

> ☹ The latest report discovered that 'nearly half the care homes for older people and younger adults, providing 210 000 places for residents, (were) still not meeting the minimum standard relating to medication.'

OK, so whose fault is it?

The NCSC say: 'The primary responsibility for this failure rests with the homes themselves.' Ouch! You'd think care homes were one of the safest places on earth, wouldn't you? Apparently not!

 So, we know there's a problem, how do we solve it? Easy:

- review policies
- monitoring the practice
- support improvement through staff training.

How? That is what this book is all about!

WHAT DO WE NEED TO THINK ABOUT?

- Privacy and dignity.
- Residents' choice and control over their own lives.
- Cultural and social, spiritual and educational needs being met.
- Health and wellbeing.
- The quality of the physical environment.
- The processes and checks in the system to deliver safe medication.

🖎 Exercise

Can you list five ways in which dependency on others impacts on residents' privacy and control over their own lives?

1

2

3

4

5

WHAT DO WE GET WRONG?

Here are the top 10 things that are most frequently messed up:

1 wrong drug was administered
2 too much medication was given
3 too little medication was given
4 medication was missed
5 medication given too late or too early
6 staff administering medication were not adequately trained
7 medication was left unattended in a communal place
8 medication was lost
9 running out of stock of a particular type of medication
10 mistakes in records of medicine administration.

The Commission for Social Care Inspection say that training and record keeping are the most important issues that we need to think about.

They say nearly half of care providers, who are required to make changes in the way they manage medicines, fail to do so within the given timeframe.

 Take time, think about this:

A woman wanted to look after the tablets and patches that the doctor had given her for pain.

The care home staff insisted that they must keep them in the clinical room and give them to her as the doctor ordered.

Unfortunately, there were times when they forgot and other times ignored her when she asked for them.

How would you prevent this from happening?

CULTURAL ISSUES

The NHS has made a strong commitment to promote ethnicity and diversity:

⧗ Exercise

What do we need to do to demonstrate that we are sensitive to residents' cultural needs in matters concerning medicine administration in homes, and how medication is administered to people from different cultures?

Exercise

Where possible service users should be encouraged to be responsible for their own medication.
What policies need to be put in place to ensure this can be achieved safely?
Think about procedures for:

- receipt
- recording
- storage
- handling
- administration
- disposal
  . . . of medicines.

SELF SERVICE

If a service user is to take responsibility for their own medication it is necessary to enable them to do so within a risk management framework.

HERE ARE SOME THINGS TO CONSIDER

- Is there a lockable space in which to store medication?
- Which suitably trained, designated care staff may, with the service user's permission, have access.
- What records are kept of all medicines received, administered and leaving the home or disposed of . . . to ensure that there is no mishandling.
- A record is maintained of current medication for each service user (including those self-administering).

☺ Medicines in the custody of a residential home must be handled according to the requirements of: the Medicines Act 1968; guidelines from the Royal Pharmaceutical Society; and the requirements of the Misuse of Drugs Act 1971, and nursing staff must abide by the UKCC Standards for the administration of medicines. So now you know!

CONTROLLED DRUGS

Controlled Drugs that are administered by staff must be stored in a metal cupboard, which complies with the Misuse of Drugs (Safe Custody) Regulations 1973.

The administration of Controlled Drugs must be witnessed by another designated, appropriately trained member of staff.

The training for care staff must be accredited and must include:

- basic knowledge of how medicines are used
- how to recognise and deal with problems in use.

☠ A HORROR STORY

At a home, which Mr X runs with his wife, he checks every prescription that arrives from the doctor and pharmacist for errors.

Because he is a registered nurse, he has some knowledge of the kind of doses that ought to be expected and the drugs that are used.

He tells of the time when he received a batch of drugs which came from the pharmacist – in the wrong dose.

The only way he knew it was incorrect was because he happened to know the higher dose pills were a different colour.

In this case it was his experience and training that told him something was wrong.

However, in many care homes medicines are administered by staff who are not nurses and do not have this experience.

Could such a mistake happen where you work?

In a care home, where the administering of medicine is not carried out by a nurse, it is questionable whether a mistake such as that would have been noticed.

If you are not a nurse and don't have the training, would you have the courage to challenge the pharmacist or the doctor?

Your answer to this question might save a life . . .

 Here's a golden rule;

**Swallow your pride before someone swallows
the wrong medication.**

If you are not sure – ASK!

THE BASICS ON ONE PAGE . . .

Drugs are received; Receipt acknowledged and logged, Controlled Drugs recorded in a Controlled Drugs register.

Nominated Manager ensures advice and guidance is available from a pharmacist with particular regard to medicines policies within the home and any medicines dispensed for individuals in the home.

Facilities for prompt review of medication on a regular basis.

Staff briefed and trained to monitor the condition of the resident on medication and know how to seek advice from a GP if they are concerned about any change in condition that may be a result of medication. When in doubt call for help.

 Consider; residents must be able to have access to patient information leaflet in drug packaging

In the event of resident's death at, or away from the care home, medicines must be retained for at least seven days in case there is a coroner's inquest.

 Consider home's policy; in appropriate instances may residents retain, administer and control their own medication? If so, ensure they are protected by the home's policies and procedures for dealing with medicines.

Develop a risk management framework, and comply with the home's policy and procedures for the receipt, recording, storage, handling, administration and disposal of medicines.

Is resident's consent to medication required? Arrange to obtain and record it. Ensure the resident is assessed as able to self-administer medication, has a lockable space (In the case of controlled drugs a double lock) in which to store medication. Ensure suitably trained, designated care staff have access (*Consider role of residents right to privacy and any permissions required*).

Ensure that medicines in the custody of the home are handled according to the requirements of the Medicines Act 1968, guidelines from the Royal Pharmaceutical Society of Great Britain and the requirements of the Misuse of Drugs Act 1971 and that nursing staff abide by the UKCC Standards for the administration of medicines.

Ensure that Controlled Drugs administered by staff are stored in a metal cupboard, which complies with current regulations and guidance issued by the Royal Pharmaceutical Society of Great Britain.

WHOSE JOB IS IT ANYWAY?

Safety is everyone's job. Not just the management or your boss. Safety is everyone's job and it is certainly your job. In the same way that you wouldn't walk past a puddle of water on the floor in a corridor, in case someone slipped and fell, so medicines management is everyone's business.

If you are used to a particular resident and know their regime and what their medication is, and you see something being done that isn't right – the wrong medication, or administered in the wrong way, or to the wrong person, or in the wrong dose, at the wrong time . . . if you are not sure:

Do something. Tell your supervisor; challenge whoever is administering the medicine. Far better to say, 'Please forgive me interfering, it's just that I know Mr Williams always has his little blue pills at around tea time. I haven't seen him have the red pills before?'

Better to be safe than sorry!

If you see the medicines storage cupboard unlocked and unsupervised – better bring it to someone's attention.

> If something doesn't seem right, the chances are that it isn't right – so be prepared to ask the question, raise the alarm and wave the flag!

And, if you are a manager of a care home it is definitely, undeniably, 24-carat gold, copper-bottomed, bet-your-life-on-it your job to:

✂ - ✂ - - - - - - - - -

. . . take all reasonable steps to ensure that at all times the
storage, administration and disposal of medicines are strictly
controlled and that safety, efficacy and accuracy are maintained.

✂ - ✂ - - - - - - - - -

👍 Got that? Cut it out and stick it on your desk, notice board or forehead, or
someplace you won't forget!

HOW DO WE GET THE MEDICINES AND WHAT DO WE DO WITH THEM WHEN WE'VE GOT THEM?

The first part of the question is easy to answer. The resident's general practitioner must prescribe for the patient. As well as filling out the usual prescription form, in the interests of best practice, they will be asked to make a further note of what they have prescribed on the home's medication register.

When the medicines arrive they must be placed in a secure place. That means the medicine store, cupboard or in some cases the medicine's room. In any event it must be locked.

> In the event of an emergency a doctor may give staff instructions over the phone – perhaps to administer a drug that is in the home's medicines store. All of the instructions should, straight away, be added to the Register by a senior member of staff and the doctor asked to sign the entry as soon as possible afterwards and certainly no later than the next visit.

Be sure that all the medicines' labels are read, carefully. Look for:

- Specific storage requirements – for example, does the medicine need to be kept in a refrigerator or in a dark place.
- Interactions with other medicines – some people, particularly the elderly, may be on multiple medications. An interaction between some medicines can make the patient very sick and can be life-threatening.
- Dose instructions – check for the frequency and the amount, such as the number of tablets to be taken at each dose. If the dose rate is not right the medicine may, at best be less effective and at worst be very dangerous.

> ☠ If the instructions are not clear or if you are not sure, ask the pharmacy or the prescribing doctor.

☺ If in doubt, ask!

 By the way. The prescribing doctor should be expected to review each resident's medications at least every six months. However, in particular circumstance a three-month review (or 12-month) might be appropriate. If in doubt, ask.

✎ Exercise

Make a list of all the residents where you work and using the '6 months guide' write down when they last had a medicines review and when they are due for the next one.

How does that compare with the Medicines Register?

WHERE SHOULD THE MEDICINES BE STORED?

Here are the rules:

- in a locked room or locked cupboard
- dry and free from moisture
- away from the light
- free from heat

. . . and

- in their original dispensed packs – just as they come from the pharmacist
- keep all foil or blister unit dose packs unopened in the original dispensed pack until the dose is given – do not decant them into bottles or jars
- do not remove labels from medicine containers.

☺ Is that what happens where you work – go and check . . .

Yes ☑   No ☒

If the answer is no – tell the boss . . .

. . . AND WHILST YOU ARE ABOUT IT

✓ Check to see if the medicines should be kept refrigerated

If they do, best practice says there should be a separate fridge, used exclusively for the storage of medicines. Not in with the eggs and bacon and matron's skimmed milk. If that is not possible:

- place the medicines in an airtight container
- place them away from food to avoid any possibility of contamination.

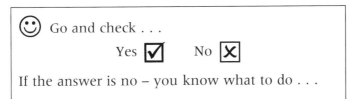 Keep a daily record of temperatures, using a maximum/minimum thermometer. Record the temperature in the Medicines Register.

> ☺ Go and check . . .
>
>   Yes ☑   No ☒
>
> If the answer is no – you know what to do . . .

SECTION TWO: ☠ CONTROLLED DRUGS

'GET IT RIGHT' CHECKLIST FOR CONTROLLED DRUGS

☒ ☑

- Keep all Controlled Drugs in a locked safe or locked cupboard.
- This store is accessible only to senior, nominated staff.
- Record all administration of Controlled Drugs in a 'Controlled Drug Register'.
- Keep a running balance of stock.
- Only nominated staff members may sign entries in the register.

🔒 WHO HOLDS THE KEYS?

Answer coming up. Read this important stuff first!

😊 Here is some good practice – to practise!

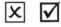 (There is no excuse for a)

- Keys to the Medicines and Controlled Drugs rooms or cupboards held by one senior staff member on each shift.
- Only one set of keys held by one person on each shift.

23

- The names of the authorised staff should be displayed so everyone knows who they are – and more importantly, who they are not!
- Access to the storage areas should be restricted to authorised staff only. So if you see someone else lurking around the stores – ask what they are doing!
- Every month, check the expiry dates on medicines and check for package damage – when medicines are constantly being taken in and out of a bottle or package they can easily get worn and insecure.
- Be like the supermarkets – rotate the stock, use the oldest first and put fresh supplies to the back.

☺ When medicines become out of date (expired) or are discontinued by the doctor, keep them in a separate, secure area for return to the pharmacy for disposal.

☺ Bottles are becoming a rare sight these days but they still exists. They are hard to damage but check them. The only damage is likely to be when delivered from pharmacist or if run over by the trolley!

But check anyway!

GET THE HOUSEKEEPING RIGHT

Errors happen easily. They happen even more easily in a muddle and mess. So to avoid errors:

- keep the medicine room or cupboard clean and tidy at all times. (Make sure it is someone's job description to do it and someone else's to check it)
- if there is a spillage – clear it up, immediately and make sure there has been no contamination with other medicines. If there has – report it straight away.

☺ An accident can happen and it is no great sin.

☹ The sin is covering up

☺ Encourage people to own up if they get something wrong. Thank them for being honest with you . . . However tempted you might be; don't bawl them out. It takes courage to own up and it takes courage to deal with problems. An environment where people can make mistakes and own up and learn from them is what helps to make airlines safe. Tell people you want to know if they have made an error, ask them how they think they could avoid making the same mistake again and reward honesty with, at least, a pat on the back . . .

Exercise

What three things will you do to encourage people who have made a mistake to own up?

1

2

3

TAKING THE MEDICINE

Remember the rights:

- right medicine
- right dose (amount and administered in the right way)
- right person
- right time.

HERE'S SOME IMPORTANT DETAIL . . .

It should all sound like commonsense but here's a Golden Rule:

☠ Never, never, never and under no circumstances give a medicine to anyone except the person for whom it was prescribed . . .

Does that sound too simple to even print?

☠ Well, it happens. It happens in day centres, care homes, residential homes and in a neighbourhood near you. People get convinced they have the same symptoms as their friend, so they try their pills! And, staff have been known to do it, with things like painkillers, when someone else gets pain.

Make sure it doesn't happen where you are! It is difficult, it is a residential home and not a prison, people are grown up and they can make choices – make sure they don't make the wrong choice. If you discover some 'pill-sharing', make sure you tell the boss.

THE RIGHT DOSE

Check prepared daily doses against the label on the container and enter them on the Medication Administration Record for signing off as the dose is administered. Paperwork – yup. It's called risk management. If the paperwork isn't done the job is not finished.

By the way; be sure to use the original dispensed container or unit dose pack to administer medicines. And, let's not forget; the resident will be familiar with a particular packaging, so it all helps to build confidence.

If this is not possible, the management must arrange a suitable alternative system which ensures that the right dose is administered to the right person at the right time. Take all reasonable steps to ensure strict control of storage and administration of medicines.

☺ During the medication round, be sure to exercise strict control over the storage and administration of medicines.

And . . .

- Except when in use, the drugs trolley and all medication should be securely locked at all times.
- During the round, when the trolley is open, never, never leave it unattended.
- The drugs round should be undertaken by two members of staff (best practice) who either have appropriate healthcare qualifications or who have been trained in dispensing medication.
- Ensure that all dispensed medications are recorded on the drugs sheet and initialled by the dispenser.

THE RIGHT PERSON

It is easy to get complacent. In a home, when you are dealing with the same people day after day, it is very easy to get content with lower standards.

However, after a long day on duty, where there are two (or perhaps more) residents with similar names and on similar medication, it is easy to get into a muddle and give Mrs White's medication to Mr White, or Mrs Whyte, or Mr Wright.

So, be sure you:

- 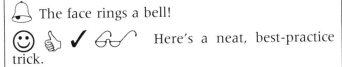 check the name of the resident against the name on the medicine container
- ask the resident to verify their name.

> 🔔 The face rings a bell!
>
> ☺ 👍 ✔ 👓   Here's a neat, best-practice trick.
>
> In places where they have it sussed they have a photograph of the resident in the medication notes. That way it is easy for an agency colleague to know who is who and easy for you to know if you are working in a large home with lots of rooms with delightful, white-haired, charming little old ladies called Mrs Smith – bless 'em! (Or Mr Smiths, of course!)

RIGHT DOSE, ADMINISTERED IN THE RIGHT WAY

Always check the instructions. Maybe, whilst you were off work for the weekend, the resident's GP has paid a visit and changed something. Unless

 Familiarity breeds errors.

you are a clairvoyant (in which case, what are your lottery numbers?) check the instructions on the packet. How is the drug administered and in what dosage?

CHECKLIST FOR ADMINISTERING MEDICINES

Always ✓

- Administer the medicines to the resident directly from the container.
- Make sure the resident has fluids to take with the medicine – ask them if they have a drink; if not, be prepared to provide one.
- Are there any special instructions to comply with?

☹ Don't accept 'Leave them there dear and I'll take 'em with my hot milk before I go to bed . . .'

Always ensure that oral medicines are swallowed. Do not leave medicines with the resident to be taken later.

✓ Make a record on the Medication Administration Record that the medicine has been administered and taken, by signing in the space provided.

☺ The sheet should also have room for you to record the fact that a dose has been withheld, refused or an extra dose given if the original dose was dropped, damaged or otherwise wasted.

HERE'S WHAT YOU DO ABOUT CONTROLLED DRUGS

When they are administered they must be recorded on the Medication Administration Record and Controlled Drugs Register, and signed for.

If for any reason a resident declines, or does not take, their medicine: remember, they are not prisoners, but they are in your care and you do have a responsibility.

So, ever so politely, ask why and then report what has happened to your supervisor and manager.

☹ The answer might be: 'Well. I just don't think they are doing me any good and they upset me.'

Sounds like time for a medicine's review!

☺ A competent patient has the right to refuse to take any medication at any time. The problems really start with an incompetent patient. No-one can give consent for someone else and the healthcare practitioner should act in the patient's best interest.

So, with a patient judged not to be competent, discuss with the doctor if the resident is refusing medication.

☠ MADE A MISTAKE WITH THE MEDICINE?

Has the wrong person got the wrong pill?
Here are two 'don'ts':

Don't panic and Don't hide your mistake!

One wrong dose may not be life and death, or it might be very serious. It depends on what the medicine was and what other medicines the resident is already taking.
There is only one thing to do:

☺ **Record and report the mistake to a senior member of staff straight away.**

Expect them to inform the doctor right away and complete an incident report.
Keep the resident under observation.

THIS IS A RESIDENTIAL HOME AND NOT A PRISON

You must expect that the resident may want to be in charge and administer his or her own medication.

In which case:

The resident should be provided with somewhere to store the medication.

A locked drawer or cupboard (A 'must' if there are Controlled Drugs involved).

There should be two keys for the store, one for the resident and one available to a senior member of staff.

Here's what you must check ✔

* The medicines, every week, to ensure they are being taken at the proper dosage. It is the residents choice, yes, that's true. But a watchful caring question; 'How are you getting on with your pills, Mrs Williams?' never hurt, or offended anyone.

> ✔ ☺ 👍 A senior member of staff and the resident's doctor must be satisfied that the resident does have the ability to take their own medicine.
>
> The position should be reviewed regularly and no later than every three months.

GOT A HEADACHE?

From time to time residents, who may or may not be on regular medication, may want some help with a headache or some other minor ailment such as constipation or a cough.

The home should have a range of household remedies to hand. They should be kept separate from residents' regular medications.

Before administering a proprietary household remedy, you must be sure that the symptom is not an indicator of something more sinister. Change in bowel habit or rectal bleeding in older people can be life-threatening, a persistent headache could be the precursor of something serious and a persistent cough that doesn't clear up after a couple of weeks is likely to need some treatment from the resident's GP.

So, always be certain to check with the resident's doctor and make sure the dose of proprietary medicine is entered in the medication register – the dose and the frequency.

☠ Even simple household remedies may combine with regular medicine to produce an adverse reaction.

☺ The residential home should establish a 'protocol' or procedure for the administration of household remedies. They should be agreed with the prescribing GP and include: a definite period of time for their use and a time when they should be reviewed by the doctor.

Oh, and if a resident is taking vitamins or any other non-prescribed items, be sure to make a note of them in the Medication Administration Record. And, to be on the safe side, make sure the GP knows – you can't be too careful with the ginseng or St John's Wort!

TAKING THE MEDICINE

There is a lot of evidence around to show that people don't take their medicines. Up and down the land, medicine cabinets of the nation are groaning with unfinished and unused pills and potions!

Why don't people take their pills? It is an important issue, even for care and residential homes where drugs are administered as part of the day to day routine. Medication cannot be expected to do its job if a course is not finished. Antibiotics are a good example.

🙁 Here are a few reasons:

- prescriptions are not collected, or dispensed
- the purpose of the medicine is not clear
- the pills 'don't work'
- side effects make the patient feel unwell
- fear that they might be dangerous
- dosage is inconvenient or the instructions may not make clear the way in which they should be administered
- a physical problem in taking the medicines, such as; opening the container, difficulty in swallowing, or problems with handling small pills
- horrible taste
- too difficult to comply with complex regimes for taking multiple medication.

🙂 Fortunately, in all of these cases, a resident in a home that has got its medicines management sorted out, can expect help.

Drugs should be administered at the right time, in the right way and residents can be helped to take them. The Home can be responsible for collecting the prescription and for making sure the medication is available and no one runs out.

⟋⟋ There is a little book (well quite a fat book actually) that is the doctor's bible for all things pharmaceutical. It is called the British National Formulary (BNF). It is interesting to read. Perhaps there is one where you work, if not ask a friendly doctor to let you have a look.

It contains all the advice a clinician might need about pills and potions. There is a very telling paragraph which is worth reproducing here:

> The prescriber and the patient should be agreed on the health outcomes that a patient desires and on the strategy for achieving them ('concordance'). The prescriber should be sensitive to the religious, cultural and personal beliefs that can affect the patient's acceptance of medicines.
>
> Taking the time to explain to the patient (and relatives and carers) the rationale and the potential adverse effects of treatment may improve compliance. Reinforcement and collaboration from the patient's pharmacist also helps. Advising the patient of the possibility of alternative treatments may encourage the patient to seek advice rather than merely abandon unacceptable treatment.

. . . and so say all of us!

> By the way, for more on that strange word 'concordance' have a look at www.medicinespartnership.org.

How do you fit into all this? Well, you sort of do, and sort of don't. It's just about making sure you know what to expect and if necessary, be able to reassure a resident. So expect the doctor or nurse to discuss, with the patient, all treatment options, very carefully, to ensure that they are content to take the medicines as they are prescribed.

Who better than care home staff, trained to administer medicines, to talk to their residents about the medicines, how they are managing them and whether there are any unwelcome, or unexpected side effects. Care home staff can be the eyes and ears of the prescriber.

☠ THESE AREN'T MY USUAL PILLS . . .

If you hear that from a patient – pay attention, close attention. You may be giving Mrs White's pills to Mrs Whitaker. On the other hand, the pills may be right – they have just been dispensed from the pharmacy in a new format.

Pills and medicines that are 'generic' medicines (that is, manufactured as the basic chemical rather than as a brand name, e.g. paracetamol rather than Panadol®) can (and often are) made by a number of manufacturers. One manufacturer may make up a drug as little blue pills whilst another may make the same drug as little yellow pills. On occasion, even the names may be different, too. All too commonly they are manufactured as round white pills which can create another problem in terms of confusing one with another!

Generic medicines are generally cheaper than the branded alternatives. In extreme cases a generic drug may be as little as one tenth the cost of a branded alternative. They are made to the same high standards and there is no difference in their make-up. GPs have targets to prescribe generic medication as one way for the NHS to manage its overall medicines budget.

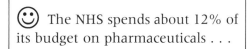 The NHS spends about 12% of its budget on pharmaceuticals . . .

QUERY FROM THE PHARMACIST?

We all know the jokes about doctors' handwriting. In these days of computerised prescription generation, the 'handwriting thing' is less important. Nevertheless, from time to time the pharmacist may have a problem or query with a prescription. What can we expect to happen?

• The pharmacist should always attempt to contact the prescriber to clarify any confusion that may exist with the prescription.
• If they do speak to the prescriber and the pharmacist is satisfied, they may go ahead and provide the medicines, even if the prescription is wrong. However, they must correct the prescription and sign it and do everything they can to ensure that the prescription is corrected and signed by the prescriber as soon as possible.
• If the pharmacist cannot contact the prescriber they may, if they are satisfied that they know what the prescription should be, go ahead. The

pharmacist must mark the prescription 'prescriber not contacted' and in any event, they may not supply more than five days' supply, or alternatively, the smallest amount available in the case of prepacked medicines.

☹ . . . however, if the pharmacist is in any doubt, the prescription must be referred back to the prescriber.

So, when a GP comes to the home and handwrites a prescription, it is worth looking at the prescription form to make sure everything the pharmacist needs to know is on the form.

Here's what to look for.

- Prescriptions must be legibly written and signed by the prescriber and can be in pen, biro or whatever, provided the finished result is indelible.
- They must be dated.
- They must have the full name and address of the patient.
- Preferably (but not necessarily) they need the age and date of birth of the patient. A date of birth is good practice and reduces the risk of error in the pharmacy.
- Where there is a potential for doubt, the sex of the patient should be added.
- The name of the drug – not abbreviated – must be shown.
- The symbol NP, on NHS forms, should be deleted if the name of the drug is to be left off the label.
- The quantity may be indicated by the number of days' treatment.
- The dose and frequency – these directions should be in English and without abbreviation. Some doctors like to show-off with a bit of Latin!

> ☺ You don't need to know this, but, hey . . . It is a legal requirement for prescription-only medicines to include the age of children under 12 years on the prescription.

> ☺ Did you know:
>
> . . . docs and dentists may prescribe medicines that are not licensed or have been withdrawn. They have to tell the patient about the medicine, why they wish to prescribe it, what the benefits and hazards are and the consequences of not using it and make a note in the patients medical history . . .
>
> Well, you do now!

- Where medication is to be taken 'as required', the minimum dose interval should be included.

- If a number of items are on one prescription, make sure that they are legible and the instructions are clear. It can be a bind to write three prescriptions for nine items, but trying to squeeze nine different drugs onto one prescription form can lead to accidents. For handwritten drugs three per form is about right.

At the surgery, virtually all doctors generate prescriptions on a computer. The fundamental rules of; *when, what medicine, how often, how much, for whom, and by whom,* still apply. It was formerly necessary to ensure that all prescriptions for Controlled Drugs were handwritten with strengths and doses in letters as well as figures. However, it's now OK to use the computer to generate the prescription but the quantity must be handwritten in *words* – not figures.

☺ The prescriber may ask the pharmacist to put a description on the label, such as: Sedative Tablets – this may be helpful for a self medicating resident.

ADVERSE REACTIONS

If you are administering medication regularly you will, perhaps, become aware of adverse reactions of drugs or their side effects. It is highly likely that the resident will tell you. Particular vigilance is required to identify adverse reactions in the elderly. They may be generally unwell and not associate a new symptom with an adverse drug reaction.

HERE ARE SOME THINGS TO THINK ABOUT

- Any drug is capable of causing an adverse reaction in any patient. The patient may have had a course of the drug previously without untoward response, so past usage is not an infallible way of knowing that there are no problems with the drug
- The drug may cause a variety of side effects or allergic reactions. Allergy may present in a variety of ways such as rash, blotchy weals (known as urticaria), vomiting, breathing difficulties, flushing or even collapse.
- Newly prescribed or purchased medication may interact with existing drug therapy causing adverse effects. This is as true for complementary therapy medication as it is for mainstream pharmaceuticals.
- Age may alter the metabolism or excretion of drugs and a smaller dose is often needed.
- Lack of familiarity with the drug or its delivery system (e.g. types of inhaler, suppository, etc.) may cause difficulties with administration.
- In very rare circumstances a doctor or nurse might warn a resident that there is the likelihood of an adverse reaction to a drug. Remind the patient and check they are OK.

☺ WHAT TO LOOK OUT FOR IN THE PATIENT

Side effects can impact on a patient in a host of different ways. It is sometimes easier to think about the effects by looking at individual body systems.

* **Gastro-intestinal effects.** Drugs may lead to such things as diarrhoea, constipation, vomiting, haematemesis (vomiting up blood) and abdominal pain.
* **Dermatological (skin) effects** such as rashes, irritation, scaling, ulceration, allergic rashes or blister formation.
* **Neurological (nerve) effects** such as headache or a feeling of being 'hungover', giddiness, disorientation, drowsiness, fainting, tingling or numbness.
* **Vascular (blood vessel) effects** such as cold fingers and toes, feeling of giddiness or faintness on standing (called postural hypotension and caused by blood pooling in the legs lowering the pressure), flushing or sweating.

Of course, virtually any drug can cause side effects and most drugs cause the most common effects such as rashes, nausea and vomiting, headache, etc. The possible side effects will all be listed on the information sheet which accompanies the pills. It is well worth taking some time to read the side effects in order to be aware of any possible reactions and to avoid any surprises.

> ☠ These are just pointers and things to consider. In every case of a possible side effect, or an adverse reaction, tell the prescriber or a doctor straight away.

41

Don't get MUDDLED UP

Some drugs have names that are remarkably similar. Don't get into a muddle.

☹ Here are some common ones that can cause confusion:

carbamazepine and carbimazole
clobetasol and clobetasone
chlorpropamide and chlorpromazine
Lamisil and Lamictal
Depo-Medrone and Depo-Provera
fluoxetine and fluconazole
Losec and Lasix
Noriday and Norimin

☺ And don't forget:

penicillamine and penicillin

Do you know the differences? Well, here are the answers:

- carbamazepine – taken orally and used in treatment of trigeminal neuralgia, some types of seizure and manic-depressive psychosis
- carbimazole – treatment of an overactive thyroid
- clobetasol – steroid used in **potent** steroid ointments and creams
- clobetasone – steroid used in **moderate** steroid ointments and creams
- chlorpropamide – a drug to treat diabetes
- chlorpromazine (Largactil) – drug used for sedation and in the treatment of schizophrenia, psychoses and mania

- Lamisil – a drug used as a tablet and in cream as an antifungal
- Lamictal – a drug used in the treatment of seizures
- Depo-Medrone – a steroid used for injections into inflamed joints
- Depo-Provera – an injectible long-acting contraceptive
- fluoxetine (Prozac) – treatment of depression and obsessive compulsive disorders
- fluconazole – an antifungal used in the treatment of thrush
- Losec (omeprazole) – used in oesophageal reflux, duodenal and gastric ulcers
- Lasix (frusemide) – a diuretic
- Noriday – a progesterone-only oral contraceptive (which can be used for women who should not be given oestrogen)
- Norimin – a combined oral contraceptive containing progesterone and oestrogen
- penicillamine – drug used in the treatment of rheumatoid arthritis and can also be used in lead poisoning
- penicillin – an antibiotic.

SECTION THREE: MEDICINES MANAGEMENT

Here, in more detail, are all the issues about medicines management. Take you time to read through the sections and complete the exercises, with colleagues, as an aid to learning and then online for your accredited learning.

MEDICINES RECORD

There are several references, in the book, to 'the medicines record'.

It is at the heart of medicines administration. Everything you need to know. What medicine, how much, when and by whom administered.

Later in this section there is an image of what a medicines record looks like. It is taken from the records that are supplied by the pharmacist, Boots. Most pharmacists will provide a similar record sheet. However, the one we reproduce is clear, comprehensive and is how it should be done! Well done Boots.

A medicines, or medication record at the very least, should include all the following information:

Name of patient ✓
Date of birth ✓
Address – that is the room or suite number ✓
Allergies ✓
The doctor's name ✓

So far, so simple . . .
   Next you need a record of: OK ✓

- what medication
- when the course is started
- the time of administration
- the dose
- the prescriber's signature
- the 'route', i.e. oral etc.

Next, we need to know:

OK ✓

- who administered the medication
- the full record of administration over a period weeks, or the full course of medication.

. . . And, when things don't go right:

OK✓

- if the medication was refused
- medication refused and destroyed
- medication returned to the pharmacy or destroyed
- nausea or vomiting
- patient in hospital
- away on holiday, with family (sometimes referred to as social leave)
- special instructions about timing or method of administration
- a space for other notes, to record occurrences and unusual observations.

👍 ✓ ☺ For real best practice a photograph of the resident should be attached to the record. This is an invaluable idea to ensure agency or new staff don't make a mistake and administer the medicine to the wrong patient. It saves having to keep asking for verification of the patient's name. And should patients become confused – the benefits are obvious.

🔒 You must keep the records for a minimum of three years from the date of last entry, and make doubly sure they are retrievable for inspection – not stuck in the loft, or in a box in a shed and are clean and dry!

💾 ⚛ ☺ Think all this stuff should be done on computer – you're right. It will be. We are already heading in that direction. You'll be interested in looking at this: www.connectingforhealth.nhs.uk/crdb/boardpapers/all_images_and_docs/crbb/emm_report_v08.pdf.

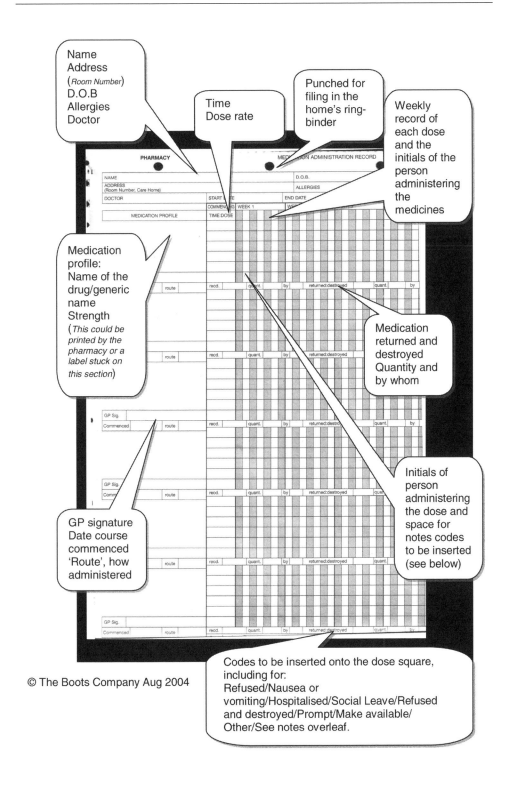

Name
Address
(*Room Number*)
D.O.B
Allergies
Doctor

Time
Dose rate

Punched for filing in the home's ring-binder

Weekly record of each dose and the initials of the person administering the medicines

Medication profile:
Name of the drug/generic name
Strength
(*This could be printed by the pharmacy or a label stuck on this section*)

Medication returned and destroyed
Quantity and by whom

Initials of person administering the dose and space for notes codes to be inserted (see below)

GP signature
Date course commenced
'Route', how administered

Codes to be inserted onto the dose square, including for:
Refused/Nausea or vomiting/Hospitalised/Social Leave/Refused and destroyed/Prompt/Make available/Other/See notes overleaf.

Where are the medicines coming from?

One of the keys to good medicines management is a good relationship with the local pharmacy.

'Local' is good, as there will be times when a quick trip to the pharmacy is what's required. However, don't sacrifice efficiency for local. A residential home of, say, 20 or more residents, most of whom could be expected to be on at least one medication (and some many more), might place quite a strain on a small pharmacy to provide the level of service that you will want.

👍 ☺ Here are some of the basics that you will definitely need. Be sure the pharmacy can offer them, this time, next time and every time.

It would be really good if the pharmacy can do all this?

☒ ☑

- It goes without saying the service from the pharmacy should be timely and accurate and able to work to deadlines and timelines.
- Can they provide advice? The administration of medicines, the contra-indication of some medicines and even the mix of medicines a resident may be taking – the pharmacist should be a sound first port-of-call for advice.
- Can they help with staff training? As the administration of medicines gets more complicated and names and packaging more confusing, a pharmacist might be a good source of basic familiarisation training for new staff, and refresher training for established staff.
- Can they deliver medicines? Is the service available for routine and urgent prescriptions?

Four ticks in the box and you have a pharmacy to die for!

👍 Also, be sure the pharmacy can supply all of the residential home's requirements, drugs and equipment.

Here's a checklist – make sure the pharmacy can do all this, no sweat, no mistakes, no messing! If they can't, no problem – find one that does!

The selected pharmacy and the residential home should be able to agree the following points. They should be written down and in the form of a protocol (That's a code of safe and correct conduct) covering, at least, the following points:

> Make sure the pharmacy service meets the needs of the resident. Remember, they live in a care home, not a prison. They should have full confidence in the home and the pharmacy to provide for their needs – just like they were living in their own home.
>
> ☺ Well, it is their own home – but you know what we mean!

	Yes	No	Fix it
• when and how the medicines and other products will be delivered			
• procedure for acquiring emergency medicines and out of hours service			
• who will deliver the medicines? Identify a nominated employee known to the home			
• a 'gold standard' would be a regular visit from the pharmacist to ensure continuing good practice, checking records and auditing medical stocks to ensure the system is running as it should			
• limit the dispensing of medicines to one month's supply only – to avoid waste and overstocking			
• make sure all medicines are correctly labelled, clearly on each container			
• ensure all medicines carry full directions for use and dose rate and carry advisory or cautionary labels where appropriate			
• ensure the medicines are in containers that are suitable for administration to individuals			

- manage the continuity of supply of medicines for residents who are for the time being away – holidays, family visits or hospital
- compile and maintain a 'medicines profile' for each resident
- carry out regular stock checks and controls and undertake the removal and disposal of damaged, discontinued and out-of-date medicines
- carry stocks of normal household medicines.

If they have got that lot right, here's some more. Ask if the pharmacy can:

☒ ☑

- provide information for the resident, the home's staff and (when necessary) the GP to make sure the patients gets the absolute best benefit from the medicines

. . . and the home should make sure that

☒ ☑

- medicines are stored neatly and in accordance with a system that all the staff understand (not just thrown in the drugs trolley or cupboard)

☠ Where a resident is prescribed more than one medicine it is very important to ensure there is no adverse reaction between each drug (or, indeed, a cocktail of drugs). How could such an event happen?

Modern pharmaceutical products are sophisticated and complicated. Doctors would expect to know about the side effects of the drugs they are prescribing and they would be expected to know about interactions between drugs in common use. Expect the doctor and the pharmacist (who is also an expert) to work in partnership; they will be able to spot the potential for an adverse interaction between drugs.

Don't forget even the best doctors are fallible and sometimes a locum, or new doctor may not be fully aware of the total picture.

Better safe than sorry. Make sure the pharmacist knows you are relying on them.

- the storage facility, room, cupboard or trolley can be adequately locked and a nominated, responsible person on each shift is the key holder
- administered at the correct dose and right method of administration.

AND TRAINING?

From time to time we all take a pill or a medicine for this and that. The GP tells when to take the medicine and the pharmacist makes doubly sure we know what we are supposed to be doing by writing the instructions on the packaging.

Here's a question for you. If a medicine is to be taken three times a day, what does that mean?

- three times a day after a meal
- three times a day, four hours apart
- three times a day eight hours apart
- three times a day; in the morning, at lunch time and before going to bed
- three times in every 24 hours?

Or, taken with a drink?

- a hot drink
- a cold drink
- a mouthful of water
- a pint of water
- a large gin-and-tonic
- dissolved in water.

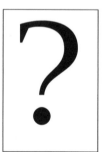

Or taken after food?

- a biscuit
- a three course lunch
- a sandwich
- a packet of crisps.

> Don't panic – here are the answers:
>
> Three times a day will usually have a specification in terms of timing in relation to food. Antibiotics for example are best taken before food. If the prescription does not say what is best, ask the prescriber.
>
> With fluid again may need clarification. Usually pills need only sufficient fluid to enable them to be swallowed but sometimes a glass of water is required. It is usually the former, unless the latter needs to be specified.
>
> After food is usually less difficult. Generally a meal or even a small snack is sufficient.

☺ 👍 If you have a good pharmacist they will be able to tell you what's what, help train staff all about handling medicines safely, storing them correctly and administering them to residents properly.

☠ ☺ 👍 Remember, as a residential home staff member, you take on the responsibility for the safety of your residents. It is essential that, at all times, residents do not make a mess of taking their medicines. If they do so, it may be serious, to be avoided and very, very undesirable. If you make a mess of their medicines it is all of the above and a good case for a lawsuit, perhaps a crime, certainly very career-limiting and something you will spend the rest of your life regretting.

☺ ☺ If you are not sure, ask, don't take chances, don't create risk and treat every resident like they were your most loved relative.

Always:

- accept only the highest standards of care for the residents
- be sure to guard the wellbeing of residents and protect fellow members of staff by ensuring all methods of medication administration and storage are as safe as they can be. If you spot something wrong – speak-up!
- be prepared to be accountable – because you are.

WRITING A PROTOCOL?

What's a protocol. Here's what the dictionary says:

> French protocole, from Old French prothocolle, draft of a document, from Medieval Latin protocollum, from Late Greek protokollon, table of contents, first sheet : Greek prōto-, proto- + Greek kolléma, sheets of a papyrus glued together (from kollan, to glue together, from kolla, glue).

. . . save that for the next time you want to look very, very clever!

However, for our purposes, a protocol means a 'code of correct conduct', appropriate and containing recognised best practice.

For a protocol to work, everyone involved should know and understand it and agree with what is in it. If everyone marches in step, sings off the same hymn sheet and does the right thing, time after time, we get a very smart group of soldiers, a fantastic choir and a safe medicines management policy!

The protocol should be available to the residents and their families or close friends, the staff, pharmacist and the responsible GP. That way everyone is in the loop and everyone knows what to expect and what to do.

> ☺ The secret of quality isn't money, the secret is consistency. Finding out what you do, deciding on whether or not you want it, then putting things in place to make sure you get it every time, time after time, until you don't want it any more. That's why you need a protocol – so you get the good stuff every time. Easy, eh?

It should describe how medicines should be stored. And, if residents are to be taking care of their own medication, the conditions under which this can be agreed.

It should include how the medicines are prescribed, who can do it (taking into account resident's consent) and the procedures for obtaining prescription drugs and the conditions under which oral instructions from the doctor can be accepted and complied with.

The protocol should include the responsibilities of staff and who has access to medicines and under what conditions. For instance, who is the medicines keyholder on each shift and their substitute in the event of an emergency (such as the nominated member of staff leaving before the shift is finished for illness or other reason).

There needs to be a clear statement of how medicines are stored, and procedures for their disposal in the event of them becoming redundant or out of date.

> ☺ If a doctor is attending a resident privately (and it is the resident's choice, after all), how does the practitioner get paid, who does it and when and how? Similarly, if prescriptions are to be paid for, what is the procedure and reimbursement detail.

The residential home should keep careful records about the medicines and who, how and when they are administered, plus any untoward incidents. This constitutes a 'medical record' and is private to the resident. The protocol should spell out who can create a record and who, other than the resident, has access to it and under what circumstance – with or without the resident's expressed consent.

Here's some more to include.

- Who takes responsibility for the key, the medicine cupboard or room and where is it recorded?
- When do they have that responsibility?
- What preparation should be made for the medicines round?
- How are medicine round records maintained?
- How are details of medicines prescribed for residents recorded?
- Under what circumstances can household remedies be administered to residents?
- How are unwanted medicines disposed of?

Answers:

 Got that? Good!

THE CHEAT'S GUIDE!

☺ Here's a quick checklist for busy residential home managers. Get a tick in the 'yes' box for all of this and you won't have too much to worry about!

It's a long list; make note of what you have to follow up on, or things you want to check out. Feel free to make copies of the list to discuss with colleagues – we are very nice people and we don't mind!

Here we go.

	Notes
1 Written policies and procedures must be in place to cover all aspects of medicines' management.	
2 The aim of the policies is to promote the safety and wellbeing of the resident and the safe practice of home staff.	
3 The ideal is to show how to best support residents in the safe self-administration of their medication.	
4 Demonstrate how staff are made aware of policies and procedures and their practice is checked.	
5 Medicines must never be used for social control or punishment.	
6 A member of staff is designated as the responsible person to supervise the safe use of medicines if residents are unable or unwilling to self-administer their medication – this is in addition to the home manager or proprietor.	

7 The responsible person should be appropriately trained and assessed as competent to undertake this responsibility.

8 The pharmacist should be known to the responsible person and the homes, management and proprietor.

9 The General Practitioner or, where there is more than one, dispensing doctor should all be known to the management and proprietor (and the GP should know how to identify the responsible person on duty).

10 Written policies must be in place to cover procedures for obtaining, storing and recording medicines.

11 Policies should cover the eventuality of specialist procedures such as PEG[1] feeds and nutritional supplements and who is qualified to administer them,

12 Records of medicines administration should clearly record who has administered the medicine and when and at what dose. The name should be clearly written and a signature appended.

13 Procedures should be in place and known to staff, if medicines are incorrectly administered.

14 Record keeping must be in accordance with Care Homes Regulations, Children's Home Regulations and the Independent Healthcare Regulations or the Regulation of Care (Scotland) Act 2001.

Notes

---

[1] PEG is short for Percutaneous Endoscopic Gastrostomy. It is a tube that passes through the abdominal wall into the stomach to allow patients to obtain food without having to swallow.

15 The registered person (the care home owner/proprietor or manager) is responsible for the maintenance of accurate, clear and precise records

16 Records should be checked to ensure they are legible and up-to-date and provide a complete audit trail of medication.

17 When completed, charts and records must be safely stored and new charts and records referenced back to their predecessor record and the originating prescription.

18 An up-to-date reference of current medication prescribed for each resident should be maintained at all times.

19 If records are kept on computer, the provisions of the Data Protection Act 1998 must be considered and appropriate advice taken and recorded.

20 The law requires residential (care) home records (not in the case of a children's home) to be retained by the home, even after the resident has left the home. Good practice is to keep the records for a minimum of three years from the date of last entry, and these records should be retrievable for inspection

21 All medicines, wheresoever they come from, such as; medicines supplied to residents on discharge from hospital, medicine prescribed in an emergency or acute episode or regular medication, brought into the home must be recorded.

Notes

22 Where a new resident moves in, some confirmation of their medication regime should be obtained. The counterfoils from repeat prescriptions are often useful.

23 This record must include: the name of the resident for whom the medication is prescribed; the date of receipt; the full name, strength and dosage of medicine; the quantity; the name and signature of the person receiving the medication at the home.

24 The means of storing the medicines should make it possible to easily identify who the medication is prescribed for.

25 Where a resident is able and wants to administer their own medication, a record should be kept of any medicines (their quantity, strength and dose), obtained and handed to them.

26 A Medicine Administration Record chart (MAR chart) must be maintained and completed on each occasion medication is administered to a resident.

27 Non-prescription medicines should be included in the record.

28 The record must show: the name and signature of the person administering the name and dose of the medicine.

29 The record must be retained and available for review, inspection and audit.

30 Staff must be instructed to check the medicines record at each administration of medication. Regular dosage should not be assumed, as fresh instructions might have been given whilst the worker was off-shift.

Notes

31 Whilst GPs are not obliged to sign a residential home's medicines records, good practice dictates the GP would sign the record when dose or medication is varied or changed or other instructions are given.

32 A record of household medicines administered by, or to a resident should be available to a GP.

33 Where a resident declines to take a prescribed medicine a record should be kept and, having regard to the resident's rights to choice and privacy, the GP should be notified.

34 Some pharmacies provide printed MAR charts. There may be a charge for this service as it is not required under the reimbursement regulations for the NHS – whilst it is the pharmacy's duty to ensure the record is accurate it does not absolve the home's responsibility to check they are accurate.

35 Ensure a complete audit trail of medicines administered in the home.

36 If medication is no longer required a record must be kept, detailing the following: date of disposal and how the medicine was returned to the pharmacy; the quantity involved; the name of the resident the medication was prescribed or purchased for; the name and signature of the member of staff who disposed of the medicines.

37 When the resident moves away from the home, to a relative, carer, or another home or hospital, a full record of medication that is taken or transferred with them should be made.

Notes

☺ Here's some technical stuff you probably don't need to know – but it will make you look very knowledgeable and super bright! And it is very interesting!

THE MEDICINES ACT

The Medicines Act 1968 covers the supply of medicines to all care homes in the United Kingdom – this was passed into law before the days of devolution and we had four national health services.

The Act identifies medicines into three categories.

- General Sales List (GSL): may be purchased from any retail outlet sometimes known as 'over-the-counter' medicines (OTC).
- Pharmacy Only (P): may be purchased from a pharmacy when a pharmacist gives their OK.
- Prescription Only Medicines (POM): only obtained on a written prescription, signed by an authorised prescriber (a doctor or a nurse).

☺ However, nothing is simple! Any of the first two medicine categories can be prescribed for – as in the third category.

Prescribed medicines are the property of the person for whom they are prescribed – and not the residential home. It is important to remember that. The home is the safe custodian of the medicines and has a duty of care to make sure they are safe and administered, with consent, in accordance with the prescriber's intentions.

It is usually a bad idea to mess about with the packs of prescribed medicines. For instance, mixing batches of

☠ All medicines covered by the Act (and for our purposes that means all of them) may only be administered to the person they are prescribed for. So it is not lawful for a home to provide medicines to a resident, using another person's medication. Medicines cannot be regarded as 'stock' or 'store' items. This includes surgical sundries, dressings and nutritional supplements that have been prescribed.

pills, or decanting them from one container to another. If you do, you could end up with a big problem with product liability.

Always use up the current packet before the new one is opened.

Some homes still use devices, sometimes called Nomads, which have spaces for each drug by time and day – they look like fishing tackle boxes. Good idea? Well . . . it is easy to get into a muddle loading them, accidentally tip the contents out or even mix up the compartments.

We don't like them. Sorry, Mr Nomad.

It does what it says on the tin

All medicines have to be supplied in safe and secure packaging. That means:

- with some exceptions, that we need not bother with, oral solid dose medicines (for all practical purposes that means pills and solid medication designed to be dissolved) come in blister packs these days. Bottles and plastic pots with child-resistant lids are becoming more and more rare
- similarly, liquid medicines. Child resistant? Where they are still in use, that means a re-closable child-resistant container (the ones with the irritating lids you have to twist or squeeze or both – that only the kids can do it!), or in so-called unit packaging in strips or the blister type.

There is an exception; if the user of the medication is unable to open the pack, in which case the pharmacist can be asked to supply the pills, or whatever, in something they can manage. Elderly and arthritic patients are an obvious example. A frail elderly person may not be able to manage to tear a strip, or push a blister pack.

Residential homes may also ask for medication to be supplied in a 'normal' (non-child-proof) container.

The label

Yes, it must have one and it must contain the following information:

- patient's name
- date of dispensing
- name and strength of medicine
- dose and frequency of medicine.

66

👍 If the medicine is in what they call a 'multiple container' – such as eyedrops in a bottle in a box, or a tube of cream in a box – the label must be on the bottle or the tube, or the jar, or whatever is in the box. That's in case the box gets thrown away and then no one can remember how to take the medication, or where to rub it in!

HERE ARE A COUPLE MORE USEFUL FACTS TO MAKE YOU LOOK LIKE A WORLD EXPERT!

The law tells us that medicines prescribed under the NHS are prescribed, individually, for each patient and that they are their property alone.

☺ Did you know it is European Law that a patient information leaflet (PIL) must be supplied with each medicine (including those supplied in monitored dosage systems) that and these should be made available to the service user?

Well, you do now!

HERE ARE SOME IMPORTANT THINGS TO LOOK OUT FOR

Make sure the GP, or other prescriber, such as a nurse, writes full instructions on the prescription. Particularly, dosage and how and when a medicine is to be taken.

Sometimes a prescriber will write what they call an 'indication' (the when and how a medicine is taken), 'as required'.

Be sure you know what that means; the dose, how often, how much and the maximum to be taken in a day.

> 👍 The National Service Framework (NSF) for older people (England) recommends home residents should have their medication reviewed every six months or earlier if the resident's needs change.

BULK PRESCRIBING

You can only do this in England and Wales. It saves a lot of paperwork and messing around, but the rules are quite strict. Bulk prescriptions may be written for medicines and dressings, including bandages. For Prescription Only Medicines (POMs), the rules are changing. Patients can now get some 'repeats' direct from the pharmacist without having to go to the doctor.

Doctors who are responsible for the NHS treatment of 10 or more residents in a care home, with 20 or more residents in total, may, in certain circumstances, issue a bulk prescription for NHS medicines and dressings for the treatment of two or more residents at the home.

This can be complicated and the residential home staff has to be on top of this. They have to know which doctor is prescribing for which patients and keep really good records.

Because it is complicated and not without the seeds of a fine old muddle, not all doctors are keen on the idea and many don't do it. Perhaps that's why it is illegal in Scotland!

☠ IN AN EMERGENCY?

The Medicines Act says that prescription only medicines (POMs) can be supplied in an emergency, at the request of a doctor and without a prescription.

So, in an extreme case, it is not impossible to imagine a situation where a resident is unwell, the doctor is consulted over the phone and he, or she, instructs the staff to give the patient a pill from the medicines cupboard that might have been prescribed for another resident. Is this legal?

WELL, IT'S ALL VERY TRICKY

Whilst this is outside the NHS regulations and seems to break all the rules and protocols, it may not be 'illegal'. However, the home should make a careful note in the medicines records and the doctor be asked to sign the entry at the first opportunity.

☺ HERE ARE THE ISSUES SPELLED OUT IN A BIT MORE DETAIL

In an emergency a doctor may need to give staff verbal instructions to provide or change medication. However, there are some complicated legal reasons why a care home may not be able to carry out these instructions. Written confirmation will be needed and a fax might just do the trick, or (perhaps) even an e-mail that has been printed out.

☠ A word of caution

A 'fax' of a prescription is not legally valid. Why? Because it isn't written in indelible ink and the fax does not have an *original* signature of the prescriber!

However, you can use a fax to indicate that a prescription exists. So, if a doctor, dealing with an emergency, indicates, in the fax, that a prescription has been written and will be produced as soon as is practicable – everyone is happy!

I know, it sounds daft, but the rule is designed to prevent a fax being used several times over – an easy thing to do when dealing with a busy pharmacy.

E-mail? Much too modern for the legal beagles to have considered. In the world of commonsense expect a printed out e-mail, electronically filed, to be treated in the same way as a fax.

By the way, medicines listed in Schedules 2 or 3 of the Misuse of Drugs Regulations 2001 must not be dispensed against a fax (Or e-mail!).

In order to avoid the legal pitfalls it is important to get this organised in advance. How the GP, or the GP's locum, or out-of-hours service, dealing with an emergency, will confirm their instructions in writing. It's back to our old friend the 'protocol'. Decide in advance what will happen and when. Record messages and phone conversations, who said what, to whom and when.

☺ . . . AND ONE MORE USEFUL THING

Where a prescription is issued and the home staff are to present it to the pharmacist for dispensing, where the resident is unable to do it for themselves, it is the job of the manager of the home, or other designated responsible person, to sign the so-called 'exemption declaration' on the back of the prescription form, on behalf of the resident.

MONITORED DOSE SYSTEMS

These are the all-singing, all-dancing repackaging systems, offered as an 'add-value' service by some pharmacy chains. Some do it for free, others charge for the service.

Medicines are repackaged in blister packs, in single doses. The packs are often colour-coded to indicate the time of day that the medicine is to be administered. Sometimes the pharmacy chain will provide a storage system for the blister packs. They are bespoke and are impossible to use with other systems – a hook to keep your custom!

Whilst these systems can be very helpful, there are some issues to think about and, perhaps discuss with the pharmacist.

- Do you want to be locked into one type of system – what are the benefits?
- These systems are only suitable for some medicines – which ones?
- When the medicines are repacked, could their expiry be affected?
- The system is not appropriate for medicines prescribed for 'as required' as they could exceed their shelf life – which ones?
- The suitability of the medication to be repacked under this type of system should be checked with, and approved by the medicine manufacturer – what is their advice?
- Tablets or capsules which look similar (and many do) and can't be identified one from another are not suitable and should not be placed together.
- Labelling should be clear and make it easy for individual medicines to be identified.

Here's a nice muddle!

It's all about something called Signed Orders.

Before the Care Standards Act 2000 and Regulation of Care Act (Scotland) 2001, the person designated the 'matron' of a nursing home was able to purchase a stock of Prescription Only Medicines (POMs), using what was called signed orders.

However, former residential care homes could not.

Then, along came the Care Standards Act 2000 and the Regulation of Care Act (Scotland) 2001. Under these two pieces of legislation it is not clear what the legal status of a care home offering nursing care is and has not been clarified in respect of the Medicines Act.

So, where stock POMs are legitimately held they may only be administered to an individual resident and where there is a written instruction by an authorised prescriber, such as a doctor or nurse.

And, by the way, just for the record, Children's Homes were not permitted to obtain POM medicines unless they were previously registered to provide nursing care such as hospices.

Got that?

OVER-THE-COUNTER MEDICINES?

We keep saying it, a residential home isn't a prison. If a resident, with all their marbles, wants to take an over-the-counter medicine, who are we to stop them?

The trick is to make sure they talk to our old friend the pharmacist.

What about the more esoteric medicines, such as homeopathy, naturopathy or herbal remedies? Well, if that's what they want – you never know it might work! Talk to the pharmacist or the GP to make sure there is no possibility of an adverse reaction with an existing medicine.

Make sure there is a care home policy about over-the-counter remedies. Keeping a small stock of the obvious things is no bad idea.

However, they shouldn't be labelled for the use of a single resident, a record should be maintained about when and who and how they are administered and, guess what, make sure there is a protocol in place!

🔒 SAFE AND SECURE STORAGE OF MEDICINES

It's all commonsense really. Remember, always, that medicines are the property of the resident – not the home. So, just like any other of a resident's property you may be asked to look after, medicines must be kept safe.

Of course there is the extra dimension that medicines, in the wrong hands, for the wrong person, at the wrong time – are dangerous. So, they are to be kept double safe.

Here is what you have to do:

If the resident is to be responsible for their own medicines then, for safety's sake, they should be provided with a lockable drawer, or cupboard. Then it's up to them to keep safe custody.

However, in the event of a resident who becomes unwell, and is in need of some medication, but who has lost or misplaced the key, then what happens?

☺ 👍 ✔ If a resident is able to visit the pharmacy and get their own prescription does this mean they are able to self-medicate? If someone is disabled and unable to get to the pharmacy does this mean they are unable to self-medicate?

The answer is no to both questions. In the ugly words of management-speak, the management at the home has to do what is called a 'risk assessment', to decide how much the resident can do for themselves and how much help they need. It's not all or nothing. Some help can contribute to dignity and independence – don't say that isn't what you will want when your time comes!

☺ Commonsense tells us that the home should have access to the medicines and that tells us a duplicate key is a good idea.

Keeping a back-up key without the knowledge of a resident is an invasion of their privacy. So, if a resident is to be 'self-medicating', make sure they understand that there is a duplicate key in case of emergencies and that the cupboard or drawer should not be used for the storage of valuables of anything other than medication. Make sure a note is kept of when the resident was made aware of the arrangements.

OK, SO WHAT HAPPENS WHEN YOU ARE IN CHARGE OF THE MEDICINES?

First things first. There must be what is called a 'designated place' that is an appropriate place set aside and agreed to be used solely for the safe storage of medicines.

Appropriate? Well, that includes being big enough, lockable and at the right temperature.

HERE ARE SOME STORAGE DO'S AND DON'TS

☑ In deciding where to store medicines, do take account of the size of the home, the number of residents and their likely, long-term need for medication and the nature of any other support they are likely to need. In most cases a drawer is out, a cupboard unlikely and a store room – ideal.

☒ Don't store medicines in a toilet, a kitchen, in a sluice room or next to a heater (or over a radiator!)

☑ Think about where to store nutrition supplements – do they require a refrigerator?

78

☑ Dressings and ostomy products can be bulky and must be stored in a warm, dry place.

☒ Always make sure medicines and other materials are stored off the floor. Nice deep shelves are ideal.

☑ Think about access to the products. High shelves and short nurses are not a good idea. Similarly, take into account bending and lifting. Make sure there is a safe-step arrangement and that the room has plenty of good lighting. Natural sunlight is not a good idea.

☒ Don't share the storage facility with any other function. Not a fuse board, a coat store, cleaning materials, or golf clubs. Just medicines and allied products only.

☒ Do not keep the keys to the medicines store on the master set of keys for the home. The lock should not be capable of being opened by the master key. The issue of keys to the medicines area should be limited to authorised people only, who sign to say they have the key at the beginning of each shift and a record kept of the handover at the end of the shift.

> 🔒 The room, store or cupboard must be capable of being locked and should be kept locked at all times.

THRILLS ON WHEELS

Using a medicines trolley? Make sure:

☑ The trolley is big enough and capable of keeping each resident's medicines separated from each other.

☑ The trolley must have a lock and must be kept locked, when unattended, particularly during a drug-round.

☑ If the trolley is used to store drugs – chain and lock it to the wall when not in use. Or, lock it away in the drugs store.

CONTROLLED DRUGS? (CDs)

The rule of thumb is keep 'em separate and keep 'em locked up. Here's some more details:

> Subject to Home Office direction, the storage of CDs where administration is undertaken by care staff should be in accordance with the Misuse of Drugs (Safe Custody) Regulations 1973 as amended. If CDs are incorporated into Monitored Dosage Systems then the whole box is subject to Misuse of Drugs (Safe Custody) Regulations.

Here's a bit more technical stuff.

☠ In homes where care staff administer medicines (as opposed to presenting them to be swallowed and such like), a Control of Substances Hazardous to Health (COSHH) Regulations assessment should be undertaken of those medicines that must be 'handled'. By that, take as an example; external applications such as steroids and cytotoxic medicines such as methotrexate.

The reason is simple enough; it is to make sure everyone understands what is required for the safe handing of these medications. Staff should be given a statement of their personal risk; what safe practices are to be followed to minimise any risks; and what to do should they come into direct contact with the medication. The statement should be in non-technical language. If English is not the first language of the care worker – consider providing a translation.

☺ KEEP COOL

Some medications need to be kept in cold storage. Not all of them are rare. For instance insulin, for the treatment of people with diabeties, should be kept in cold storage. In a care-home insulin is very likely to be in regular use.

All that is required is a refrigerator. If the fridge is kept in the medicines store, it need not be locked. If it is kept anywhere else (not the best idea), it should be kept locked.

📈 The temperature of the fridge has to be monitored daily. Use a maximum/minimum thermometer – record the findings.

☺ Be happy if the fridge has a normal range between 2 and 8 degrees centigrade. And, if it's not an auto-defrost machine – schedule regular defrost sessions and make arrangements for the temporary storage of medicines.

☹ If the fridge packs up – be sure staff know what to do. Using a fridge in the kitchen is not ideal but might do in extremis. Put the medicines in a sealed container and reserve a top shelf until the fridge is fixed. We are talking temporary – hours not days.

TAKING THE TABLETS

Helping people to take their medicines is called 'medicine administration'. As you might expect, there are some rights and wrongs.

The Medicines Act says that medicines may be given (or, as they say, 'administered') by a third party to the person they were prescribed for provided you stick to the instructions. That's just common sense.

However, each care home should have a clear procedure for the administration of medicines. That's more complex – but it's not rocket science.

HERE ARE THE BASICS

Care staff can only administer medicines if they are trained to do so.

So called, 'invasive' procedures have traditionally been undertaken by a registered nurse.

These days the majority of medicines are taken by mouth in liquid or solid dosage form, that means tablets and capsules.

Doing the 'medicines round' at a time that suits the home and staffing is a sign of a badly run home. The timing of the administration of medicines is often critical and the needs of the patient, not the convenience of the home, comes first.

Examples of invasive procedures.

- Subcutaneous injection of insulin. *(That means below the skin.)*
- Medicines administered by the rectal or vaginal route.
- Giving oxygen.
- Giving medicines through a Percutaneous Endoscopic Gastrostomy (PEG) tube.

Some medicines need to be taken with food, some in advance of food, some with water and some without. Inhalers and drops might be at altogether different timings to oral medication. The key to all this is the needs of the resident. Their needs, privacy and dignity should be observed at all times.

No THANK YOU!

Residents are not prisoner – they can say 'no' to their medication. If they do, and they are competent to make the decision, apart from charm and persuasion – there is nothing you can do.

However, if the resident is unable to make proper (informed) decisions, perhaps through the onset of dementia or other illness, it all gets very tricky.

If a resident says 'no', make a note of it in the medicines record and try and give a reason, if possible. (Too hard to swallow, bad taste, gives indigestion, doesn't do any good etc.) Discuss the reasons with the prescriber or the pharmacist. Perhaps the drug comes in another format that is easier to ingest or tolerate.

If all this fails, the relatives or carers need to be involved, along with the care staff and the doctor.

☺ Sometimes the wellbeing of the patient will dictate that some subterfuge in the administration of the medicine is commonsense.

Disguising the medicine in a drink or food might be an option.

It should be done with everyone's agreement (home management, doctor, relatives etc.) and a full record made in the resident's notes. It is good practice to create a written policy around what has been agreed, so that everyone is aware of what is happening and how it is happening.

✎ Under the Regulation of Care (Scotland) Act 2001 details of any instance in which medication is administered to a service user without the consent of the service user or a person duly authorised to consent on their behalf must be notified to the Care Commission.

☠ You might be tempted to crush a tablet and dissolve it to make it more palatable. Check with the pharmacist or the manufacturer (most pharmaceutical companies have helpline numbers on the patient information leaflet that comes with the packaging) to make sure the tablet isn't coated to delay its absorption. Crushing it might have a bad effect for the patient in terms of the therapeutic effect of the medicine.

When administering a medicine (horrible phrase), helping a resident to take their medication (better), never remove the drugs from the original container – the one they were supplied in from the pharmacy.

Always take them out of the packet, in front of the patient, check the name with the patient and the name of the medicine and the dose – you can, then, for hygiene purposes, place them in a dish, or pot.

☹ Never take a medicine out of its container and give it to a colleague to administer – all sorts of risk and confusion could be involved.

POLICY, WHAT POLICY?

A care home must have a written policy for the administration of medicines. That way everyone knows what they are supposed to be doing – including Agency and other temporary staff.

Here's the basics of the policy – be sure and cover these issues as a minimum.

Done ☑

1 The resident/patient's identity to be checked to ensure the correct medicine is administered.
2 Staff to check the patients, the name of the medication and the dose.
3 Staff to be made aware of recent changes in medication.
4 Always check the medicines chart against the pharmacy label.
5 Always check that the name of the resident, the name of medicine, strength, and number of dose units and frequency match.
6 If there is any mismatch check with the duty manager or the pharmacy before administering the medicine.
7 Check how the medicine is administered.
8 Staff administering the medicine will sign the administration record immediately after the medicine has been given.
9 Where the home uses medicines administered from a MDS system containing more than one medicine, staff administering the medicines

must be able to distinguish each individual medicine and be aware of any specific instructions, e.g. with water or before or after food.

10 Make a record of medicines that are declined or refused – include the reason.

11 When the prescription allows for a choice in dose (one or two tablets) record what is administered.

12 Record the name and signature of the member of staff administering the dose.

13 Record the date and time.

In addition:

☑ The home should have a record of the staff authorised to administer medicines and a sample signature, or initials.

☹ Some homes will accept the initials of staff administering medication. This could be open to abuse, error and confusion and is not best practice but many Medication Administration Records don't leave any space for much more than initials. Make sure they are identifiable and distinctive.

☠ **If something goes wrong?**

It is essential that the home has a written policy instructing what must happen if a medicine is administered in error.

Likewise for situations where there is a problem with any aspect of medicines delivery.

☺ 🏖 OFF TO THE BEACH?

✈ When a resident goes on holiday or away for a few days, they will want to take their medication with them. Give it to them in the dispensed containers (Do not decant them into envelopes or 'handy little boxes'!). Make a note in the home's records and be sure the resident and or the carer/relative knows the dose and administration regime.

☺ 🩳 ✉ And remind them to send you a postcard!

Perhaps the resident is regularly away – attending a daycare centre or class (they do you know – have a life!) and needs to take medication whilst away.

Think about asking the pharmacist or doctor if the administration regime can be changed to save taking the medicines away from the home.

If that isn't possible, ask for a supply in a separate container that the resident can take with them and self-administer.

✓ And make a note in the medication records.

WHEN YOU DON'T NEED THEM ANYMORE – THE MEDICINES, NOT THE RESIDENT!

Remember the medicines belong to the resident and not the home. So, if the resident has had enough of your stunning and loving care and wants to move – they should take their medicines with them.

If the resident recovers and no longer needs the medication, with their consent, take it back to the pharmacy for safe disposal.

☒ Don't flush them down the loo!

1 If you look on the packaging you will see that all medicines have an expiry date. When they get out of date agree with the resident that they should be sent to the pharmacy for disposal.

In all cases of disposal – be sure and record it in the home's medicine's record.

☹ When a resident dies, from whatever cause and in whatever circumstances, hang on to their medication for at least seven days in case the Coroner's Office, Procurator Fiscal (in Scotland) or the courts want them.

RESIDENTS WHO NEED OXYGEN AND YOU?

Whilst working in a care home it is highly likely you will come across residents who will depend on a supply of portable oxygen.

There have been problems with the new system of supply and it is better you know a bit about how the system works than know nothing about it and find yourself in the middle of some medical crisis or huge row.

So, we think it is worth a few pages to bring you up to speed.

OXYGEN

To help with respiration some residents may need a supply of oxygen. Sometimes temporarily and sometimes for much longer periods. It used to be that a GP would write a prescription for home oxygen and it would be fulfilled at the local pharmacist.

☹ Recently there have been changes – groan. A new system to take your breath away!

Whilst GPs are still (for now) able to write a prescription for the pharmacists, the new system involves outside contractors who supply the gas. There's the problem.

There have been a couple of well-publicised cases where patients appear to have been left without a supply of oxygen. The finger of suspicion has pointed to the contractor.

> 😐 If it ain't broke don't fix it. Why did the government change the system for the supply of medical gases?

Indeed, some GPs have been so concerned about the situation that they have called upon the government to go back to the old system. They describe the handover to the contractors as 'chaotic'.

The Pharmaceutical Services Negotiating Committee, which represents community pharmacists in the NHS discussions, warned there was a 'risk the chaos of the handover period would continue long-term'.

This is not the time or the place to debate the rightness of the policy – that's for you and your colleagues at the next tea break! However, it is important that you know there are problems with the system. So, you need to know exactly how the new system works and what to expect –

> ☹ The Royal Pharmaceutical Society said the government had 'failed to implement the change-over in an organised manner'.

> ✎ . . . pharmacists were only reimbursed for supplying oxygen until 31 July 2006.

and what to look out for to make sure your residents don't get left breathless!

THE NEW SYSTEM IS ALL DONE ON THE HOOF

The HOOF replaces the old FP10 ordering form.

The HOOF stands for:

Home Oxygen Order Form

The resident's GP will order oxygen for short-term and short burst oxygen needs and palliative care.

The GP fills in the HOOF and once issued it will remain valid until requirements change.

That means the order will keep being repeated, to ensure a continuous supply.

✔ ☞ ☠ The first job is to check that supplies are continuous. If there is any sign of a delay

☺ Patients with long-term needs will be assessed by respiratory consultants – the GP will arrange this.

It's all a bit of a LTOT – no, not the Italian State Lottery!

New residents who require long-term oxygen therapy (LTOT) will be referred for specialist assessment by a specialist team, but the GP can prescribe for the patient whilst waiting for the assessment to take place.

or a breakdown in the supply chain – tell the boss. If you are the boss – tell the GP.

Most of the private companies have helplines. Ask the GP practice to tell you what the number is and stick it on the wall where the medicines are stored and where everyone can see it. If there is a problem – don't be afraid to call for help.

Because the suppliers of the oxygen are 'outside' the NHS, patients must sign a HOCF! Gets worse doesn't it? A HOCF (or should that be 'an HOCF'), is a Home Oxygen Consent Form. It must be completed when the first HOOF is issued.

To help the prescriber, there is detailed guidance on the back of the HOOF on how to fill the form in. That easy, eh?

☒ There is a tick box on the HOOF (Box Number 14) relating to the supply of an oxygen conserving device – the box should only be ticked if the device is *not* wanted – all nice and confusing, eh?

😬 Because the NHS lives in the world of cutting-edge technology the HOOF is faxed to the supplier, to the Primary Care Trust and to the Trust Clinical Oxygen lead. Yes, all three . . .

A copy of the consent (HOCF) should be given to the patient and both the HOCF and the HOOF should be scanned into the patient record. The supplier should send an order acknowledgement and that has to be scanned into the patient record, too!

In an emergency expect the HOOF to be completed but the order phoned to the supplier. Bear in mind the emergency HOOF will remain in place until the regular HOOF (if there is one) supersedes it.

The various consent and other forms can be downloaded from www.primarycarecontracting.nhs.uk/118.php.

> ☹ So, let's see what this means in the real world: Dr Boggs comes to your home, writes up a HOOF for a resident, Mr Williams, and gets him to complete a HOCF – there is no blanket provision for care homes. He then legs it back to the surgery where he sends off the order to the supplier Gasses-R-Us, makes the scan of the HOCF for the practice records and then rushes back with the HOCF for Mr Williams. You, then, might make a copy for your records.
>
> If you can think of a more clunky procedure, please let us know!

☠ Some practices are warning their GPs that emergency HOOF supplies are very expensive and, if they think an ongoing supply is indicated – they should fill-in a regular HOOF at the same time.

☺ If a resident goes on holiday and a supply of oxygen is required – a new HOOF should be completed – but don't forget to cancel it when the holiday is over.

The whole system is based on the premiss that oxygen, once ordered, will keep turning up in the same quantities, until someone tells the contractor a change or cancellation is needed. If no one tells the contractor – expect a big lorry to turnup, or not . . .

To find out more try: www.primarycarecontracting.nhs.uk/118.php.

At the time of writing this book the contact details for the various contractors are as follows – but bear in mind, over time the contracts may change hands and the information could get out of date:

Supplier and Region	Freephone Number
Allied Respiratory (Medigas): SW & SE London, Thames Valley, Hants and IOW, Surrey & Sussex	0500 823 773
BOC: Eastern England	0800 136 603
Linde Gas: North East	0808 202 0999
Air Products: North West, Yorkshire & Humberside, East Midlands, West Midlands, North London, South West	0800 373 580

Copies of the forms can be downloaded from:

www.primarycarecontracting.nhs.uk/120.php

British Lung Foundation have a very helpful Helpline on:

08458 50 50 20

and their web-address is:

www.lunguk.org

. . . that's it. Now go and catch your breath!

THE SYSTEM AT A GLANCE

☺ PATIENT NEEDS OXYGEN				

Long term	Ambulatory	Short burst	**Emergency short burst**	Oxygen prior to hospital discharge

L-T & Ambulatory O_2 should not normally be prescribed without a Respiratory Consultant assessment unless for example for Palliative Care

Emergency short burst:

1. Call supplier to initiate supply.

2. Complete Patient Consent Form (HOCF)

3. Complete HOOF, stating it is confirmation of the telephone order

4. If oxygen is needed beyond 3 days, complete a second HOOF at the same time, stating when the routine oxygen supply commences and the emergency supply should cease.

5. Fax HOOF(s) to supplier

6. Take 3 photocopies and send to PCT, GP and Respiratory Team

7. Original HOOF and consent form stays on patient record

NB: An emergency oxygen prescription supply (4 hour response) costs 9 times more than routine supply, and will continue for a minimum of three days and then until cancelled or a routine HOOF is received.

Long term / Ambulatory:

1. Complete Patient Consent Form (HOCF)

2. Complete HOOF

3. Fax HOOF to supplier

4. Take 3 photocopies and fax to PCT, GP and Respiratory Team

5. Original HOOF and consent form stays on patient record (scan)

Oxygen prior to hospital discharge:

Wherever possible request at least 3 days before discharge. In this case:

1. Complete Patient Consent Form (HOCF)

2. Complete HOOF

3. Fax HOOF to Supplier

4. Take 3 photocopies and send to PCT, GP and Respiratory Team

5. Original HOOF and consent form stays on patient record

For 'next day' response tick same in Box 11.

Otherwise proceed as Emergency Short Burst Oxygen.

In both cases a second HOOF to initiate the routine provision will need to be completed and processed as above.

1 **When to use the HOOF**   ☒ ☑

   The HOOF replaces the FP10 prescription for
   oxygen and is required for all patients who use
   home oxygen cylinders from 1 February 2006.
   [Concentrator patients who do not use cylinders
   do not need a HOOF.] Ambulatory or long-term
   oxygen should not normally be ordered without
   prior assessment by a consultant respiratory
   physician.

   Complete a Home Oxygen Consent Form
   (HOCF) at the same time as the HOOF to
   obtain patient consent for sending the order to
   the supplier as they are 'outside' the NHS.

2 **Completing the form**

   The form must be completed in full – omissions
   are likely to result either in delay in supply or a
   call from the supplier for clarification. Please
   note.

   • Prescribers must confirm that patient consent
     has been obtained using the HOCF (tick box).
   • Modality of supply (boxes 7–9 on the HOOF)
     – sufficient information (e.g. flow rate, hours
     usage) should be given to allow the supplier
     to provide the most appropriate modality for
     the patient. In general, for short burst oxygen
     therapy 2 litres/min is an appropriate flow
     rate unless the patient has been assessed by a
     respiratory physician and an alternative flow
     rate suggested.
   • The tick box relating to an oxygen-conserving
     device (box 14) should be ticked only if a
     device is *not* wanted.

3 **Emergency oxygen and out-of-hours supply**

   Call supplier on out-of-hours number to initiate
   a supply within 4 hours. Complete the HOOF
   and HOCF as above and fax the HOOF to
   supplier as confirmation of the order as soon
   as possible. If ongoing oxygen is needed
   (beyond 3 days), complete a second HOOF so

that supplier knows when the emergency supply ceases and the ongoing supply begins.

4 **Completing the order**

Fax the HOOF to the supplier on the dedicated fax line. They will inform the patient about installation.

Three copies of the form are required. *The form is not available in a carbon-copy pad, so it will need to be photocopied.* Send by safe haven fax or courier marked 'private & confidential'.

- copy to the relevant PCT in which the patient's GP is based
- copy to the patient's GP record
- copy to Respiratory Specialist Team.

Original HOOF stays with the patient's record.

5 **Holiday provision**

Patients should ask their GP to complete a HOOF for oxygen required while they are on holiday (within the UK). Include the duration of supply and oxygen delivery address in box 13.

SOME STUFF ABOUT MEDICINES

This is probably not 'must-know knowledge' but we think it's interesting so we have inflicted it on you. We have a sneaking suspicion that you'll like it, too!

☕ COFFEE TIME READING, QUIZ AND UNBRIDLED ENJOYMENT!

Let's start with some 'Fascinating Facts'.

How many prescriptions do you think are dispensed annually? To give you a clue we've given you the numbers for 1950 and 1990

- 1950: 217 000 000
- 1990: 360 000 000
- 2001:
- 2004:

Answers: 2001 – 588 000 000 and 2004 – 686 138 500.

In other words . . .

Prescription volumes are speeding up. In the period 1996–2000 the average rate of increase was 3% each year. By 2000–2004, the rate of increase was 5%.

Any ideas why?

There are probably three reasons.

- Wider choice of drugs.
- More conditions treatable.
- Clinical guidance lays down standards for prescribing.

New, NHS National Service Frameworks are aimed at a number of treatment regimes and patient groups. They make treatment and care protocols more explicit. The use of prescription medicines is part of the Frameworks and will account for some of the increases in prescribing.

Second, the new General Medical Services contract, the new way of paying GPs, will have something to do with it.

As a result of the contract, part of a GP's income is now based on the number of points they achieve in a year. The points are linked to certain aspects of care.

This includes the diagnosis and management of conditions in patients who, perhaps, were previously unaware that they might need help. Heart disease and diabetes are just two examples of conditions that GPs are now encouraged to look for and treat. This pushes up the drugs bill.

Third is a move away from the old 30-day prescriptions to prescriptions written up for 28 days. This is a minor change but it will have had an impact.

And finally, the general increase in demand for healthcare.

How much do you think the average prescription costs? That is the cost of the pills, not how much the patient actually pays (or is exempt from paying) in prescription charges.

We've given you a start:

- 1990: £6.66
- 2001/2:
- 2004 (England):

Answer: 2001/2 – £10.65; 2004 – £16.16.

 By the way; in 1950 it was the equivalent of 16p!

WHEN DID YOU LAST HAVE A PRESCRIPTION?

The nation seems to be able to swallow its way through a incredible number of pills and medicines. It is a truly awesome amount! Some folk go for years without ever seeing a doctor, never mind taking medicines.

But, there are formidable number that don't!

Do you know the average number of prescriptions, per person (England) per year?

Have a guess. Is it:

☑ Put a tick in the box

☐   3

☐   5

☐   7.7

☐   8.3

☐   13.7

Answer: 13.7

☺ All doctors have targets to write a certain number of prescriptions using generic medicines. In 2004 they managed 74%!

99

☠ FROM TIME TO TIME THINGS GO WRONG

What are the most common causes of prescription error?
  First, things go wrong in the administration department!

- Prescriptions are written for the wrong patient.
- Sometimes it's the wrong or inappropriate drug.
- The wrong dose or frequency is written on the prescription.
- Communication breakdown/failure to notify side effects.
- Patients are not properly followed up or monitored.

Next there are clinical errors. Here are some examples.

- Overlooking a patient's allergies.
- Cosmetics, e.g. photosensitivity, depigmentation.
- Side effects, bleeding, migraine, rash, etc.

There are other areas of risk.

- The so-called Primary/Secondary Care Interface. This is where a patient has been in hospital and been prescribed for. On their return home, into the hands of primary care, misunderstandings can occur and misprescribing might be an unwelcome outcome. This has the potential to work the other way round.
- Repeat prescribing errors are not uncommon and good doctors are always very cautious about repeat prescribing arrangements.
- Over- or under-use; patients taking the wrong amounts of medication.

- Failure to adequately monitor patients who are on long courses of medication.
- Failure to review medicines. Over time a patient's needs and condition can change. It may mean a change in medication

Sometimes it goes wrong, right from the start. There are errors in the prescription. It does no harm to make sure that all the boxes are ticked!

☑ Heading – Surname, one forename, address, date of birth and age.

☑ Drug name – ideally generic.

☑ Dosage – milligrams. *Other units in full, with decimal parts written like this: 0.125 mg.*

☑ Total quantity.

☑ Usage clearly specified.

☑ Any empty space deleted.

> ☺ At the end of the day, when all is said and done, when it's all over and all the rest of it (!)
>
> **Clinical responsibility for prescribing rests with the practitioner signing the prescription.**

How often does it all go wrong?

Probably more often than you think . . .

The right phrase is 'medication errors'. What's one of them? Here's the definition:

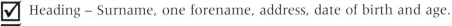

A medication error is a *preventable error* that may cause or lead to *inappropriate medication* or *use* or *patient harm* while the medication is *in control* of a *health care professional*

How many? In the United States a study suggested prescription errors cause harm in ~1% of patients (Bates 1995, *JAMA*). In the UK a study published in the *British Medical Journal* in 1999 suggested similar findings . . . ouch.

There are lots of reasons for error. Here are the most common:

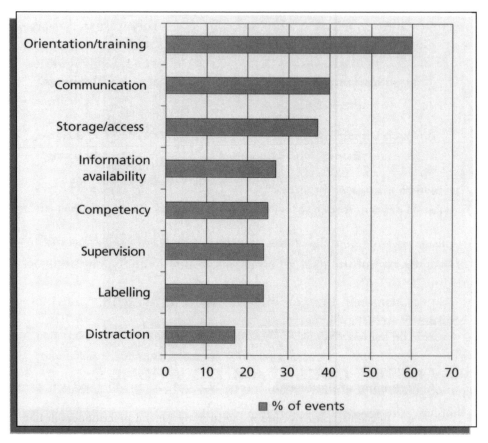

Source: NPSA 2003.

As you will see, a lot of errors can be associated with parts of care that are not directly attributable to doctors and prescribers getting it wrong.

Food for thought!

OK, coffee break over, back to work! How many questions did you guess right?

SOME THINGS TO THINK ABOUT

These are questions, not about what you do, but about the procedures where you work. How many ticks in the box do you get? If you don't get many perhaps you need to think about bringing the issues up at the next meeting?

1 Are issues about medication and medication administration a feature of the home's complaints procedure?

2 Are the complaints routinely monitored, audited and action taken?

3 Have errors in the administration of medication resulted in serious incident reports and what action is taken?

4 Are written policies and procedures for medication administration adhered to?

5 What procedures are in place for staff to raise concerns and worries about medicines administration?

6 Is the obtaining of medication well managed?

7 Are prescriptions fulfilled and made available in a timely manner?

8 Are the arrangements for medicines storage secure?

9 Are good records kept?

10 Are the procedures for the administration of medicines adhered to?

11 Are the procedures for the disposal of unwanted medicines understood and adhered to?

12 Are residents who wish and are able to self-
   administer medicines supported and discretely
   monitored?

13 Are staff supported and trained in medicines
   management and administration?

14 Is the management of Controlled Drugs secure?

15 Is each resident's medication regularly reviewed
   by a GP?

16 Do staff have written policies and procedures for
   the administration of medication?

17 Are they regularly trained, tested and checked
   in the procedures?

18 Are staff encouraged to raise issues of medicines
   management that might be wrong?

SECTION FOUR: MORE INTERESTING STUFF!

More on Controlled Drugs

Stuff you need to know

When Controlled Drugs are administered it should be witnessed by another designated appropriately trained member of staff.

The training for care staff must be accredited and include:

- basic knowledge of how medicines are used
- how to recognise and deal with problems in use
- the principles behind all aspects of the home's policy on medicines
- handling and keeping good quality records.

✓ The receipt, administration and disposal of Controlled Drugs must always be recorded in a Controlled Drugs register.

> **What is a 'Controlled Drug'?**
> . . . in the UK, a preparation subject to the Misuse of Drugs Regulations 1985.
>
> These drugs are divided into five schedules covering import, export, production, supply, possession, prescribing, and appropriate record keeping.
>
> The first schedule deals with drugs such as LSD and cannabis for which medical prescription is not available. (Acknowledging that presently there are clinical trials in connection with the use of cannabis derivatives as a pharmaceutical preparation.)
>
> The strictest schedules for prescribed drugs are 2 and 3 and these include opioids, stimulants and most barbiturates.
>
> ☺ Now you know!

⧗ Think about this:

A care home is just that: it is a home, not a hospital and not an institution. Just like you, at your home, from time to time there will be a minor 'medical incident' like a cut finger, and the occasional headache, requiring an aspirin.

 Here's what should happen in a care home:

- First aid, treatment for a minor illness and any medication given at the home (other than by a doctor, dentist or registered nurse) must only be given by a competent designated member of staff (that might mean a qualified first-aider).
- Be sure that there is a written record kept of all treatment, medication and the nature of any first-aid treatment. The record should include the name of the person giving the 'treatment', and the date, time, medication/treatment (make sure the dosage is included) and why the treatment has been administered. The entry must be signed.

☺ Care home staff are not jailers and have no power to insist that a resident takes their medicines – or consents to treatment.

If the resident says; 'No thanks':

Keep a record of when and why medicines are not administered or are refused.

☎ Most importantly, if a resident frequently refuses medication, make sure the GP is informed.

Exercise

Make a list of the reasons why a resident might refuse medication.

For each reason, consider what action you should you take?

😊 Did you know?

- 82% of older people in care homes have a long-standing illness.
- 48% have two or more chronic conditions.
- 38% of people aged 75 and over take at least four prescribed medicines.

. . . well you do now!

Here's something you may not want to know!

 The Commission for Social Care Inspection say:

- 12% of care homes for older people, (that means about 1500 homes across the country), did not meet the medication standard
- 43% were assessed as almost meeting the standard
- 44% met the standard
- only 1% exceeded it.

For some reason homes in London and the West Midlands were doing significantly worse than other regions, while the South East was performing significantly better than the rest.

> 😐 What is it like where you work – which group do you fit into?

Homes owned by Local Authorities were found to have significantly different scores from other homes, with relatively few (9%) failing to meet the standard outright but only 34% meeting it.

Here are some of the reasons why homes fell short of the standards required.

> ✎ Exercise
> Think about why there should be such marked regional difficulties? Why should the management be different, is the availability and quality of staff an issue?
>
> What would you do to try and bring the homes up to a higher and more universal standard?

- Medicines stored insecurely or at the wrong temperature.
- Wrong medication given to service users.
- Poor recording of medicines received and administered.
- Inappropriate handling of medicines by untrained staff.

Here's what the good places looked like.

- Staff well trained and supervised.
- Medication regularly audited.
- Good working relationships with local health professionals such as GPs and pharmacists.
- Active involvement of residents in planning their care and medication.

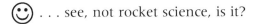 . . . see, not rocket science, is it?

GETTING IT RIGHT CHECKLIST

	Yes, doing it now	Don't do it	Need to get it organised
1 Do errors in the administration of medication result in serious incident reports?			
2 Are written policy/procedures for medication available?			
3 Arrangements in place to ensure the continuity of supplies of prescribed medication for residents.			
4 Medication storage complies with appropriate regulation.			
5 Full and complete records kept.			
6 Procedures for administration of medication documents and staff appropriately trained.			
7 Procedures for disposal of unwanted medication.			
8 Policies in place to support residents who wish to self-administer medication.			
9 Training for all care workers in the safe handling of medication.			
10 Management of Controlled Drugs in accordance with regulations.			
11 Regular review of medication by resident's GP.			

WASTE DISPOSAL

Why would a book on medicines management have a section on waste disposal? Isn't it a waste of time?

The answer is simple enough. Part of the job of managing or administering medicines could involve you in disposing of unwanted medicines or so-called sharps. What are sharps? This sort of thing:

- metal hypodermic needles
- needles with fixed syringes
- razor blades
- stitch cutters
- glass ampoules
- scalpels

✎ . . . in fact, things used in the administration of medicines or care, that are sharp.

☺ Not rocket science.

You may not be the one using the sharps but it is highly likely they will be used in the working environment of a care or residential home.

There will be other waste material, too – used dressings and the like. Here's a brief look at the dos and don'ts of waste disposal.

Waste disposal depends on what you have to dispose of, which in turn reflects the sort of residential facility we are dealing with.

The Environmental Protection Act 1990 places a duty of care to sort waste, store it safely in a suitable container and arrange for its safe disposal.

> ✎ Make a note
> Waste disposal basic requirements.
>
> - Have a written practice waste disposal policy.
> - Arrange for safe transportation and collection of waste and safe disposal in accordance with legislation.
> - If in doubt, regard waste as clinical.

There is a requirement to document disposal routes (Environmental Protection (Duty of Care) Regulations 1991). Depending on the activities conducted in the home, waste must be segregated into clinical, non-clinical, special waste and sharps.

- Non-clinical waste is material such as paper, plastic, old Tesco receipts, betting slips etc.
- Clinical waste is contaminated by blood or other body fluids.

👍 If in doubt classify the waste as clinical and dispose of it accordingly.

Clinical waste must be transported in UN-approved rigid containers. Yes, that is UN as in United Nations, (Carriage of Dangerous Goods (Classification, Packaging and Labelling) and Use of Transportable Pressure Receptacles Regulations 1996).

☺ Sharps containers are bright yellow, often with a red top and conform to UN standard 3291 and British Standard 7320, and should never be filled more than three quarters full. That way someone shoving a needle into a sharps container doesn't get stabbed for their trouble.

Sharps must be contained in sealable UN-type approved 'sharps' containers to BS 7320.

Clinical waste and sharps must be collected by authorised persons and documentation of the waste content provided and records of transfer held by both parties. Transfer notes may cover repeated transfers up to one year. You must keep the documentation for two years – and then dispose of it as non-clinical waste (even though it's about clinical waste!) Got that?

Special waste is prescribed medicines and other waste classified as irritant, harmful, toxic, carcinogenic or corrosive. This is all dealt with in the Special Waste Regulations 1996. The one you will be most concerned with is prescribed medicines – under most circumstances, they go back to the pharmacist for them to worry about.

WASTE DISPOSAL CHECKLIST

	Yes	No	Will be sorted	By whom?	By when?
• Are you aware of the different types of waste and the requirements for the correct disposal of each?					
• Is practice waste correctly categorised, stored and disposed of?					
• Is clinical waste stored in appropriate containers?					
• Are staff trained in its disposal					
• Do staff only handle clinical waste when using heavy duty rubber gloves?					
• Are systems in place for the correct transfer of waste?					
• Is waste collected by an authorised person?					
• Has the home checked the certificate of registration of the waste remover?					
• When clinical waste is removed is a signature obtained by the home?					
• Are transfer notes kept for two years?					
• Are 'sharps' sealed in UN-type approved containers?					
• Does the home ever create special waste?					

DOS AND DONT'S AT A GLANCE

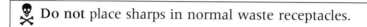

☠ **Do not** place sharps in normal waste receptacles.

☑ **Do not** resheathe, bend, break or manipulate needles by hand. Discard them intact.

☑ If there is a need to resheathe a needle, make sure that needle guards are available.

☑ Place sharps immediately after use in an approved sharps bin or receptacle; they are puncture-resistant and leak-proof.

☑ Containers for sharps disposal must be located in the work area at the point of use.

☑ Containers for sharps disposal must be closed (lid or cover closed and sealed with tape) and identified for waste collection when they are no more than three quarters full. Never overfill or force items into these containers.

☑ Report and record all injuries involving sharps.

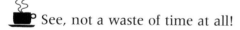 See, not a waste of time at all!

SECTION FIVE: NUTRITION

⏀ WE ARE WHAT WE EAT . . .

In February 2006, the National Institute for Health and Clinical Excellence www.nice.org.uk published guidance called *Tackling the Problem of Malnutrition in the NHS*.

Apparently, 10% of the over-65 population are malnourished and 60% of pensioners admitted to hospital have a nutrition problem.

The guidelines said that all hospital inpatients, on admission, and all outpatients at their first clinical appointment should be screened.

👍By 'screened' they meant they should be weighed, measured (for height) and have their body mass index (BMI) calculated.

Now, here's the important bit. They also said:

> . . . people in care homes should be screened on admission and where there is clinical concern.

OK, a residential home is not a care home, and neither is it a hospital. However, there are issues about the duty of care that a residential home might have, and there are issues about keeping an eye on people and making sure they are OK.

People who decide to make their lives in a residential home are unlikely to be young and they certainly won't be getting any younger. It is not inconceivable that, as they get older, eating and nutrition drop off the top spot in their agenda.

Loss of weight and eating poorly are obvious detractors from wellbeing and the healthy enjoyment of life.

There are other risks, too. Here are a few:

- compromised immune function
- increased risk of respiratory disease
- digestive disease
- cancer
- osteoporosis
- increased risk of falls and fractures.

☺ Here's the question: Is it appropriate to include a couple of pages, in a book like this, about nutrition and measurement?

If you think the answer is; 'yes', read on. If you think the answer is; 'no', tear the pages out and put them on the bottom of the parrot's cage!

If you are a 'yes' person, here we go!

WHAT IS BODY MASS INDEX?

In simple terms it is the ratio of fat in your body to the rest of your body's weight. Calculating body mass index, or BMI, is a simple way to find out how much of your body is fatty tissue and how much is muscle, bone, and other healthy tissue.

The higher the BMI number, the 'worse' it is. Well, sort of. There are people who do not agree that BMI calculations are reliable and many who believe that they are not reliable enough in connection with measurements for the young, athletes and the elderly. Well, be that as it may. The nice people at NICE have decided that it is the measurement they want to use. Who are we to argue?

In general, a BMI of over 25 contains too much fat. A BMI of 30 or more is considered obese. More important for us, in the consideration of elderly people, a BMI of less than 18.5 is not good. Indeed it puts the resident in the 'malnourished' department.

EXTRACT FROM NICE'S GUIDANCE

> Nutrition support should be considered in people who are malnourished, as defined by a BMI of less than 18.5; unintentional weight loss greater than 10% within the last 3-6 months, or a BMI of less than 20 and unintentional weight loss greater than 5% within the last 3-6 months.

HOW IS BMI CALCULATED?

The idea is to measure the height to weight ratio.

Here's an example:

Let's say you weigh 120 pounds and you are 5'5" tall.

Step one: Take your weight and multiply that by .45 to convert it to kilograms.

Answer = 54 *kilograms*. ✓

Step two: Convert your towering 5'5" of height into inches.
[5 x 12] + 5 = 65 inches. ✓

Now we have to turn the inches into metric, or meters . . .

Step three: Multiply 65 inches by the magic number .0254, which gives us 1.65 meters.

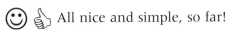 All nice and simple, so far!

Step four: Here's the clever bit: Multiply your height in meters by itself:
[1.65 x 1.65] = 2.725 *meters* ✓

Final bit: Divide the *meters* into the *kilograms*.

54 *kilograms*
2.725 *meters*

And the answer is 19.81. ✓

That means the body mass index or BMI is 19.81. Nice and healthy!

 Exercise

Go and find a calculator and find out what your BMI is, for real!

With a resident's consent it should be possible to perform this calcula-tion – indeed you can show them how to do it for themselves.

There is a quicker way! There are hundreds of websites that will do it for you. Google 'BMI Calculator' and see what you get. To save time, here's one: http://nhlbisupport.com/bmi/bminojs.htm.

Here's another one that is worth a look, because it factors-in age: www.halls.md/body-mass-index/av.htm.

☺ Just a thought: In the elderly it is often better to have a BMI between 25 and 27, rather than under 25. If a resident is older than 65, for example, a slightly higher BMI may help protect them from osteoporosis.

In the United States, in April 2005, the government issued statistics on obesity. They included this passage:

> . . . although it is clear that being overweight can have fatal results, for the elderly being underweight also appears lethal.
>
> The new study found 34,000 more deaths than expected among the underweight and most of these deaths were among people age 70 or older.

. . .interesting, eh?

In case you don't have access to the internet – here's a quite useful chart.

Body Mass Index Table

Height (Inches)	Normal						Overweight					Obese										Extreme Obesity														
BMI	19	20	21	22	23	24	25	26	27	28	29	30	31	32	33	34	35	36	37	38	39	40	41	42	43	44	45	46	47	48	49	50	51	52	53	54
	\multicolumn{36}{Body Weight (pounds)}																																			
58	91	96	100	105	110	115	119	124	129	134	138	143	148	153	158	162	167	172	177	181	186	191	196	201	205	210	215	220	224	229	234	239	244	248	253	258
59	94	99	104	109	114	119	124	128	133	138	143	148	153	158	163	168	173	178	183	188	193	198	203	208	212	217	222	227	232	237	242	247	252	257	262	267
60	97	102	107	112	118	123	128	133	138	143	148	153	158	163	168	174	179	184	189	194	199	204	209	215	220	225	230	235	240	245	250	255	261	266	271	276
61	100	106	111	116	122	127	132	137	143	148	153	158	164	169	174	180	185	190	195	201	206	211	217	222	227	232	238	243	248	254	259	264	269	275	280	285
62	104	109	115	120	126	131	136	142	147	153	158	164	169	175	180	186	191	196	202	207	213	218	224	229	235	240	246	251	256	262	267	273	278	284	289	295
63	107	113	118	124	130	135	141	146	152	158	163	169	175	180	186	191	197	203	208	214	220	225	231	237	242	248	254	259	265	270	278	282	287	293	299	304
64	110	116	122	128	134	140	145	151	157	163	169	174	180	186	192	197	204	209	215	221	227	232	238	244	250	256	262	267	273	279	285	291	296	302	308	314
65	114	120	126	132	138	144	150	156	162	168	174	180	186	192	198	204	210	216	222	228	234	240	246	252	258	264	270	276	282	288	294	300	306	312	318	324
66	118	124	130	136	142	148	155	161	167	173	179	186	192	198	204	210	216	223	229	235	241	247	253	260	266	272	278	284	291	297	303	309	315	322	328	334
67	121	127	134	140	146	153	159	166	172	178	185	191	198	204	211	217	223	230	236	242	249	255	261	268	274	280	287	293	299	306	312	319	325	331	338	344
68	125	131	138	144	151	158	164	171	177	184	190	197	203	210	216	223	230	236	243	249	256	262	269	276	282	289	295	302	308	315	322	328	335	341	348	354
69	128	135	142	149	155	162	169	176	182	189	196	203	209	216	223	230	236	243	250	257	263	270	277	284	291	297	304	311	318	324	331	338	345	351	358	365
70	132	139	146	153	160	167	174	181	188	195	202	209	216	222	229	236	243	250	257	264	271	278	285	292	299	306	313	320	327	334	341	348	355	362	369	376
71	136	143	150	157	165	172	179	186	193	200	208	215	222	229	236	243	250	257	265	272	279	286	293	301	308	315	322	329	338	343	351	358	365	372	379	386
72	140	147	154	162	169	177	184	191	199	206	213	221	228	235	242	250	258	265	272	279	287	294	302	309	316	324	331	338	346	353	361	368	375	383	390	397
73	144	151	159	166	174	182	189	197	204	212	219	227	235	242	250	257	265	272	280	288	295	302	310	318	325	333	340	348	355	363	371	378	386	393	401	408
74	148	155	163	171	179	186	194	202	210	218	225	233	241	249	256	264	272	280	287	295	303	311	319	326	334	342	350	358	365	373	381	389	396	404	412	420
75	152	160	168	176	184	192	200	208	216	224	232	240	248	256	264	272	279	287	295	303	311	319	327	335	343	351	359	367	375	383	391	399	407	415	423	431
76	156	164	172	180	189	197	205	213	221	230	238	246	254	263	271	279	287	295	304	312	320	328	336	344	353	361	369	377	385	394	402	410	418	426	435	443

Source: Adapted from Clinical Guidelines on the Identification, Evaluation and Treatment of Overweight and Obesity in Adults: The Evidence Report.

SECTION SIX: HAND HYGIENE

✋ **WASH YER HANDS!**

Ok, ok, we know. It's not medicines management. Yup. You're right.

BUT

. . . it is a huge problem. People die because other people don't wash their hands. Is that you?

You are looking after residents, many of whom will be frail and vulnerable. Good hygiene is vital, crucial and life-and-death important.

☺ SO, AS WE HAVE YOUR ATTENTION – HERE WE GO!

Sam Lister, health correspondent of the Times Newspaper, in March 2006, wrote:

> More than a third of NHS hospitals and other health trusts are unable to provide their staff with hot water, soap, alcohol rubs and other basic hygiene requirements whenever they need them, according to a national survey.
>
> A poll of more than 200 000 employees, conducted by the Healthcare Commission, has revealed alarming shortfalls in NHS hygiene, supposedly a key priority for the Government in its attempt to reduce hospital-acquired infections.
>
> The survey found that one in four members of staff felt that the trust they worked for did not do enough to promote the importance of cleaning hands to staff, patients and visitors.

127

😧 Ouch! This is serious stuff and a sombre criticism of NHS establishments. What is it like where you work? Maybe it's not the NHS but is it any better? Do you have?

- Access to plenty of hot water, soap, alcohol rubs and other basic hygiene requirements whenever you need them?
- Enough support to promote the importance of cleaning hands to staff, patients and (very important) visitors.

. . . you should have!

😦 ✓ ☠ **Why does any of this matter?**

Hospital-acquired infections, such as methicillin-resistant *Staphylococcus aureus* (MRSA) and *Clostridium difficile*, have been connected with a growing number of deaths in recent years, prompting a crackdown on poor hygiene.

A total of 7212 cases of MRSA bloodstream infection were detected in English hospitals in 2004–05. That could mean up to 300 000 infections are picked up in healthcare settings every year, causing 5000 deaths and costing the NHS as much as £1 billion.

In the Health Commission survey:

- only 61 per cent of respondents, said that their trusts had hot water, soap, alcohol rubs and paper towels available at all times.
- only 28 per cent reported high levels of hand-cleaning equipment, and one in five NHS workers said that they never had access to such facilities.

😦 It gets worse! A total of only just over half (51%) said that they had received training, learning or development about infection control in the past 12 months. That means half did not!

So, what's the answer? Wash your hands – please!

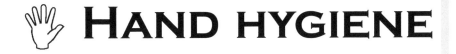 HAND HYGIENE

WE ALL KNOW WASHING OUR HANDS IS A GOOD IDEA — SO WHY DON'T WE DO IT?

The simple answers are; it is not convenient and there is confusion over what to use to clean our hands.

But it's important! It really, really is!

When to wash?

- When hands are visibly dirty or contaminated with proteinaceous material or are visibly soiled.
- Wash hands with either a non-antimicrobial soap and water or an antimicrobial soap and water.
- If hands are not visibly soiled, use an alcohol-based hand rub for routinely decontaminating hands.

> ☺ Here's a history lesson – It'll make you seem very wise!
>
> In Vienna in 1846, there was one Dr Ignaz Semmelweiss who worked in the maternity wards. He was a sharp dude and noted that the mortality rate in the wards cared for by physicians and medical students were as much as three times greater than those wards where care was provided by midwives.
>
> The problem was; the students were coming straight from the pathology lab without washing their hands. Disgusting! They were carrying infections from the laboratory to the patients. He implemented a handwashing protocol.
>
> Bingo! The mortality rate dropped to less than 1%. Result!

Antimicrobial-impregnated wipes or towelettes can be considered as an alternative to washing hands with a non-antimicrobial soap.

🖐 HERE'S HOW THE ROYAL COLLEGE OF NURSING TEACH THEIR MEMBERS TO WASH THEIR HANDS — PROPERLY!

Take off your wristwatch and any bracelets and roll up long sleeves before washing your hands (and wrists).

1 Wet hands under running water.
2 Apply liquid soap and rub hands together to make a soapy lather.
3 Away from the running water, rub the front and back of hands. Massage all the finger tips properly including the thumb, the web of the fingers, around and under the nails. Do this for at least 10 seconds.
4 Rinse hands thoroughly under running water.
5 Dry hands thoroughly with either a clean cotton towel, a paper towel, or a hand dryer.
6 The cleaned hands should not touch the water tap directly again.
7 The tap may be turned off by using the towel wrapping the tap or outlet or after splashing water to clean the tap or outlet or by another person.

. . . Not too difficult?

Good advice, thank you RCN!

 By the way:

- Towels should never be shared.
- Used paper towel should be properly disposed of.
- Personal towels to be reused must be stored properly and washed at least once daily. *Better still, have more than one towel for frequent replacement.*
- Rub hands with a 65–95% alcohol solution to disinfect the hands when handwashing facilities are not available.

✔ While alcohol hand gels and rubs are a practical alternative to soap and water, alcohol is not a cleaning agent. Hands that are visibly dirty or potentially grossly contaminated must be washed with soap and water and dried thoroughly. Alcohol is not a substitute for hand washing.

☺ Remember: Hands must always be cleaned before direct contact with patients *and* after any activity or contact that contaminates the hands, including following the removal of gloves.

IT'S IN YOUR HANDS!

Make sure you:

- keep nails short, clean and no nail polish – save that for your days off . . .
- keep artificial nails for time off, not at work
- avoid wearing wrist watches and jewellery, especially rings with ridges or stones
- cover any cuts and abrasions with a waterproof dressing.

Is this OK where you work? It should be:

1 hand washing facilities available and easily accessible in all patient areas, treatment rooms, sluices and kitchens

2   basins in clinical areas have elbow or wrist lever
    operated mixer taps or automated controls
3   basins provided with liquid soap dispensers,
    paper hand towels and foot-operated waste bins
4   alcohol hand gel available at 'point of care' in all
    care settings (So says the National Patient Safety
    Agency (2004)).

☹ If you can't give four ticks you should bring any lack of facilities, or in the wrong place, to the notice of your manager, or boss.
    👍 You have what is called a duty of care to patients and yourself and must use the facilities provided to prevent cross infection.

THAT'S THE WASHING — WHAT ABOUT THE DRYING?

If you don't dry your hands properly, you can re-contaminate them and undo all the good the washing has done! Wet surfaces transfer organisms more effectively than dry ones and inadequately dried hands are prone to skin damage.

Good quality disposable paper hand towels are just the thing to ensure hands are dried thoroughly. Hand towels should be conveniently placed in wall mounted dispensers close to hand washing facilities.

🖐 GLOVES?

Not a substitute for hand cleaning . . .

Gloves should be worn whenever there might be contact with blood and body fluids, mucous membranes or skin that is not intact. Put them on immediately before you do what ever it is that you have to do and then take them off as soon as the procedure is complete.

Discard the gloves safely and then wash your hands.
    👍 Did you know there are all sorts of gloves to chose from?

• Nitrile or latex gloves should be worn when handling blood, blood-stained fluids, cytotoxic drugs or other high risk substances.
• Polythene gloves are not suitable for use when dealing with blood and/or blood and body fluids, in other words, in a clinical setting.

- Neoprene and nitrile gloves are good alternatives if you are sensitive to natural rubber latex.

DISPOSAL?

Waste bags should be colour-coded:

- yellow bags for clinical waste
- black bags for household waste
- special bins for glass and aerosols
- colour-coded bins for pharmaceutical or cytotoxic waste.

☺ Make sure everyone knows which is which!
From time to time you may be involved in clearing up spillages of blood or body fluids, such as after someone has vomited. This is a job that has to be done right!

Once again, here's the advice that the RCN give their members – it's very sensible!

☑ Spillages should be dealt with quickly, following your workplace's written policy for dealing with spillages.

☠ Under no circumstances should specimens be left on windowsills or placed in your pockets.

☑ The policy should include details of the chemicals staff should use to ensure that any spillage is disinfected properly, taking into account the surface where the incident happened – for example, a carpet in a patient's home or hard surface in a hospital.

☑ Collecting, handling and labelling specimens. A written policy should be in place for the collection and transportation of laboratory specimens.

The RCN say you should:

- be trained to handle specimens safely
- collect samples (wearing protective clothing) in an appropriate sterile and properly sealed container
- complete the form using patient labels (where available) and check that all relevant information is included

- take care not to contaminate the outside of the container and the request forms
- ensure that specimens are transported in accordance with the Safe Transport of Dangerous Goods Act 1999
- make sure specimens are sent to the laboratory as soon as possible.

INDEX

consistency, protocols 56
containers
  see also packaging
  'multiple container' labelling 67
  pharmacists 51
contamination 25
continuity of supply, pharmacists 52
Control of Substances Hazardous to Health
  (COSHH) 80
Controlled Drugs (CDs) 10, 23–43, 80,
  107–11
  basics 12, 13
  checklist 23–4
  defining 107
  keys 23–4
  MAR 31
  Register 31
  register 107
  training 107
  witnessing 10, 107
COSHH *see* Control of Substances Hazardous
  to Health
costs, prescriptions 98
crushing tablets 84
CSCI *see* Commission for Social Care
  Inspection
cultural issues 7–8, 36

death, residents 12, 88
dentists, prescribing 38
Depo-Medrone 43
Depo-Provera 43
dermatological (skin) side effects 41
descriptions
  medicines 39
  prescriptions 39
dignity, residents' 5
disguising medicine, administering
  medicines 84
disposal
  hand hygiene 133–4
  medicines 52, 88
  waste 113–16, 133–4
distraction errors 102
diversity, promoting 7–8
dos and don'ts

storage 78–9
waste disposal 116
dose
  errors 100
  instructions 17, 54–5
  monitored dose systems 73–4
  right 28
  'three times a day' 54–5

e-mail prescriptions 71
emergencies 16, 70–2
  oxygen 95–6
  pharmacists 51
  POMs 70
  protocols 72
Environmental Protection Act (1990), waste
  disposal 113
errors 25–6
  allergic reactions 100
  defining 101
  dose 100
  familiarity 30
  monitoring 101
  numbers of 102
  prescriptions 100–2
  Primary/Secondary Care Interface 100
  reasons for 102
  reviews 101
  top ten 6
ethnicity, promoting 7–8
'exemption declaration', prescriptions 72
expired medicines 24, 88
  see also disposal

familiarity, errors 30
faxed prescriptions 71
first aid 108
fluconazole 43
fluoxetine (Prozac) 43

gastro-intestinal side effects 41
General Sales List (GSL) 64
generic medicines 37, 99
getting it right checklist 112
ginseng 34
gloves, hand hygiene 132–3
'gold standard', pharmacists 51